MW00574740

"In an unpretentious, transparent, conversat[...]
warn and instruct. Traditional, truncated '[...]
are not merely inadequate, they can be spiri[...]
Cycle blends biblical insight, educational t[...]
powerful conceptual framework that has [...]
same for yours."

Ralph E. Enlow Jr., president of the Association for Biblical Higher Education

"In our training course to help camp leaders create their own Bible study curriculum in Latin America, we discovered very few resources to help people apply Scripture. The Elmers' Learning Cycle revitalized our 2020 version of both teacher and student editions. Their book provides abundant insights for helping people obey truth, whether found in God's Word or any subject matter. Driven by a passion to close the gap between hearing and doing, the Elmers include practical strategies like asking students to do a *barrier analysis* by asking, 'What obstacles might you encounter if you obey this truth? How can you prepare to overcome them?' Their style of writing engages the reader, intertwining deeply personal experiences with insights from brain research and the social sciences. This book also crosses cultures perfectly."

Lisa Anderson-Umaña, director of leadership development with Christian Camping International, Latin America

"I am very pleased you are holding *The Learning Cycle* by Muriel I. Elmer and Duane H. Elmer in your hands. My guess is you are a teacher, whether in a formal vocational setting, or as a parent, Sunday school teacher, or business leader. You know that the operation of teaching and mentoring is a complex one. How does one person ever hope to communicate with others given the challenges and influences each listener has pressing in on his or her heart and mind, and so conditioned by culture and circumstance? Drs. Muriel and Duane Elmer bring decades of study and experience to help readers of this book learn to be maximally effective in the high and holy craft of teaching. They model these things in their own lives. I know. I've worked with them in the past and have seen firsthand how effectively and empathetically they nurtured their students across a wide range of cross-cultural settings. In fact, I have been a beneficiary of their work. I recommend this book to you knowing that they are the 'real deal,' and their book will inspire you to reach your students in an effective way."

Jerry Root, author of *C. S. Lewis and a Problem of Evil*, professor at Wheaton College

"Duane and Muriel Elmer are extremely gifted at helping ministry leaders grow to their full potential. This resource is practical and truly transformational if you apply what they are suggesting. My own ministry has been forever shaped by their insights. I'm so grateful that they have made this resource available so many more people can benefit from their experience and wisdom."

Mary T. Lederleitner, author of *Women in God's Mission* and *Cross-Cultural Partnerships*

"*The Learning Cycle* provided the foundational principles for training and motivating twenty-one hundred Rwandese church members and over a thousand short-termers from Saddleback and also undergirded the strategy for change that made their Western Rwanda HIV Initiative so successful."

Gil Odendaal, former global director of the HIV/AIDS Initiative at Saddleback Church

"Muriel and Duane Elmer have been trusted, wise guides to teachers, shepherds, and leaders around the globe for many years. The love of God and his kingdom fuels their endeavors including this volume. *The Learning Cycle* is a culmination of their life's work, sharing the wisdom they have gleaned from years of study, teaching, and service. A must-read for Christian educators."

Deborah Colwill, associate professor of educational and leadership studies at Trinity Evangelical Divinity School

"In the recognition of common grace, this book blends current research in social sciences and neuroscience with decades of teaching experience and theological reflection as it seeks to help Christian practitioners understand how to improve their teaching. It will be especially useful for theological educators who tend to have had little exposure to this kind of educational training and wish to develop as reflective practitioners. It was especially encouraging to see the final chapters on the topics of habit and character."

Marvin Oxenham, director of the International Council for Evangelical Theological Education Academy

"Why is it that the vast majority of what we are taught is soon forgotten? Why is education most often ineffective? Why do we assume that emotions are divorced from cognition? The Elmers make a strong case for teaching that leads to deep learning because it is initially meaningful and continues through the learning cycle toward the full development of the learner. They uniquely make the case for life-changing learning, supported by recent research in neuroscience, the social sciences, Scripture, and their own compelling stories as teachers. My hope is that this book will stimulate a gracious revolution of transformative teaching for thousands of educators."

James E. Plueddemann, author of *Teaching Across Cultures,* former director of SIM International

"If you want to critically reflect on how your teaching may lead students toward integrated life learning, the Elmers are here to help. They offer practical research findings and application within this renewed presentation of the Learning Cycle certain to elevate any Christian educator's craft."

Michael A. Ortiz, international director of the International Council for Evangelical Theological Education, associate professor of intercultural studies at Dallas Theological Seminary

"The publication of *The Learning Cycle* occurs in the context of challenging times for education and educators. Around the world, some question the value of education; others demand tangible results from educators and their institutions. With this current reality facing education, it is propitious for teachers to consider the nature and purpose of teaching and learning. Should teaching limit its focus to the transfer of information, insights, and knowledge to students, or should it seek to achieve transformed habits of thinking and doing in leaners? *The Learning Cycle* by Muriel Elmer and Duane Elmer is a substantive resource for educators wrestling with this question. It is required reading for anyone longing for teaching and learning to produce more than recall of information or mastery of insights."

Tite Tiénou, dean emeritus, research professor of theology of mission, and Tite Ténou Chair of Global Theology and World Christianity at Trinity Evangelical Divinity School

"If you are an educator who cares that learners live out the truth you teach, this book is for you. Whether you teach as a pastor, teach children or adults, in Christian higher education or theological education—anywhere people want to learn—this book shows how your teaching can lead to the goal you so much desire. What sets this book apart are the learning tasks the authors provide at the end of each level of the Learning Cycle, providing a promising pathway to becoming a more skillful teacher."

Miriam Charter, retired associate professor of intercultural studies at Ambrose University, former director of PhD in Educational Studies at Trinity Evangelical Divinity School

"From their vast personal experience as educators to the current science of neurobiology and educational psychology, the Elmers unlock the mystery most teachers face in the classroom—student transformation. Focusing on how learners learn rather than how content is delivered, the Elmers walk the reader through steps assured to foster the renewing of the whole person. This book is a must-read for any serious educator who is committed to students' holistic transformation."

David Sveen, president of the Domanada Foundation

"Duane and Muriel Elmer's passion for transformative and lifelong learning is prudently interwoven in their version of the Learning Cycle as clearly delineated in this book. It is noteworthy that *The Learning Cycle* includes the affective side of learning, the intentional naming of barriers to learning, and the integration of God's Word to life, critical stages that are missing in other versions of the Learning Cycle. I was introduced to the framework when I was their student and found it to be very helpful when explaining the how and what of transformative learning. I have used it since in my teaching opportunities, incorporating it in curriculum discussions and in teachers' professional development workshops both in theological education and the local church. Every time it is offered, the Learning Cycle brings the aha of discovery. My sincere appreciation to Duane and Muriel Elmer for now putting the framework in a book so that more educators can benefit. I highly recommend this book and this valuable educational framework!"

Joanna Feliciano-Soberano, academic dean at Asian Theological Seminary, Overseas Council regional director for Southeast Asia

"Muriel and Duane Elmer have combined insights and lessons from their distinguished careers as teachers with some of the most current findings from neuroscience to produce a book that helps the reader become a better educator. They do so in ways that promote better cognitive understanding, changes in behavior, and growth in Christian maturity. Written in a relatable style and incorporating stories from their experience, they explain and illustrate how we can all become more effective in teaching for life change."

Evan Hunter, vice president of ScholarLeaders International

"From more than fifty years of shared teaching wisdom and experience, Duane and Muriel Elmer take us inside the Learning Cycle to expand our understanding and expertly unpack its implications for all of us engaged in the educational enterprise. Along the way, they offer tested insights from the social sciences and those freshly available from the exploding field of brain science. This is an *essential* read for novice and experienced educators alike."

Dave Conner, director of talent development at Duke University

"*The Learning Cycle* is a marvelous integration of recent medical understanding of how the brain works and what that means for teaching and training. Building on eight decades of teaching, Duane and Muriel Elmer provide this insightful guide in which they wonderfully demonstrate a deep understanding of the craft of teaching and a commitment to continual growth as they practice the craft. This will serve as an excellent tool to use with anyone serving in a teaching or training role—in ministry, business, education, and the like. I am already utilizing insights I gained to improve my own teaching and training, and offer my highest commendation for their work. Two thumbs up!"

Scott Moreau, academic dean and professor of intercultural studies, Wheaton College Graduate School

"I received this book as I was leaving to teach Majority World pastors and missionaries. My new minilectures with open-ended questions were met with joy! But it wasn't until the groups shared that I realized the level of openness, transparency, and integration of the material taking place. The Holy Spirit was working, and conclusions were reached beyond what I had even suggested. It was worth changing my ways. Thank you, Muriel and Duane, for providing this resource that will help us good teachers and professors become much more effective. The material is engaging, providing the right amount of brain research to convince while showing us how to make the necessary practical changes to accomplish our goal as teachers—transformed students."

Ron Kuykendall, St. Andrew's Church, Gainesville, Florida

"Elmer and Elmer are experienced educators who have learned all the steps and approaches that are essential to transformative teaching, and they share them here, clearly and winsomely. *The Learning Cycle* is a terrific resource for any educator who wants to remember that great teaching is always about teaching the whole person, not just an academic subject."

Christina Bieber Lake, professor of English at Wheaton College, author of *The Flourishing Teacher*

The
Learning
Cycle

Insights for Faithful
Teaching from Neuroscience
and the Social Sciences

MURIEL I. ELMER
and DUANE H. ELMER

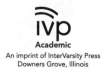

IVP
Academic
An imprint of InterVarsity Press
Downers Grove, Illinois

InterVarsity Press
P.O. Box 1400, Downers Grove, IL 60515-1426
ivpress.com
email@ivpress.com

InterVarsity Press® is the book-publishing division of InterVarsity Christian Fellowship/USA®, a movement of students and faculty active on campus at hundreds of universities, colleges, and schools of nursing in the United States of America, and a member movement of the International Fellowship of Evangelical Students. For information about local and regional activities, visit intervarsity.org.

Cover design and image composite: Cindy Kiple
Interior design: Daniel van Loon
Images: business pie chart with arrows: © Fireofheart / iStock / Getty Images Plus
         human brain illustration: © Ukususha / iStock / Getty Images Plus

ISBN 978-0-8308-5383-0 (print)
ISBN 978-0-8308-5530-8 (digital)

Printed in the United States of America ∞

Library of Congress Cataloging-in-Publication Data
A catalog record for this book is available from the Library of Congress.

P	25	24	23	22	21	20	19	18	17	16	15	14	13	12	11	10	9	8	7	6	5	4	3	2	1
Y	41	40	39	38	37	36	35	34	33	32	31	30	29	28	27	26	25	24	23	22	21	20

TO OUR MOTHERS

Mary Sophie Danielson

Ruby Lorene Elmer

Whose love, encouragement, faith, and
prayers have guided our lives

Contents

In Gratitude

*T*his book represents our more than fifty extraordinary years together teaching and learning. During all those years we sat at the feet of a host of teachers and mentors, both past and present, who prodded our thinking and challenged our assumptions. To them we owe a great debt.

We can name only a few:

Ted Ward, who showed us best practices, exposed us to the best literature, and pushed us to new horizons—all the while creating in us an unquenchable thirst for "We can do it better."

The hundreds of students and workshop participants who critiqued our Learning Cycle, asked where it was written, and went on to use it in their own teaching careers.

Miriam, Bas, and Scott, whose letters of recommendation paved the way to a publishing contract.

Fred Van Dyke, who chose to experiment with the Learning Cycle in his Sunday school class and help his learners actually practice Jesus' words in Matthew 6.

Those willing to persistently plow through our first draft, or sections of it, and make it substantially better: Lisa Anderson-Umaña, Marie-Claire Weinski, Sherry Bohn, Mary Macaluso, and Laura Van Vuuren. We are also grateful to Cheryl Warner for her editing, Dave Conner for resources, and Valerie Umaña Anderson for timely material.

Friends who over the period of a couple of years forwarded countless resource ideas for us to explore and strengthen our writing.

Al Hsu, our editor, who graciously shepherded *The Learning Cycle* to publication; and Evelyn and Breanna for their indexing.

And finally, a host of prayer warriors who faithfully prayed for wisdom and clarity as we went to our computers each day—good friends, colleagues, family members, and a small group of Thursday morning praying sisters: JoAnn, Carol, Diane, and Judy.

With gratitude we thank you for believing in us. Above all, we thank our heavenly Father, who in his mercy made it possible for us to write this book.

CHAPTER ONE

Laying the Foundation

I have no greater joy than this, to hear of my children walking in the truth.

3 JOHN 4 (NASB)

Our task in ourselves and in others is to transform right
answers into automatic responses in real life situations.

DALLAS WILLARD, *THE DIVINE CONSPIRACY*

AFTER LAUNCHING my four-year teaching career in a Bible college in South Africa, I (Duane) was invited back ten years later to speak at a conference. It gave me opportunity to reconnect with former students. Moses (his real name) would be the first. I was looking forward to it because I had poured myself into my classes and thought that, for a first-time faculty member, I had done a credible job.

We met over a delicious meal of curry and rice. I asked Moses how he was. He rehearsed how God called him away from managing an automobile dealership to our Bible college and then to ministry. All went well until after graduation. Things had gone badly for him in the pastorate. His son, a police officer, was killed in public for undetermined reasons, and other family tragedies followed. He left the ministry. In spite of all this, he was now a successful insurance salesman but sour on God, the church, and Christianity.

"So, what went wrong, Moses?" I asked, feeling overwhelmed by the tragedies and now his fragile faith.

"I don't think my Bible school education prepared me for church ministry or the problems I would be facing." He spoke without anger or criticism, just the facts as he saw it.

The jarring reality hit me: As one of his teachers, I had failed—and, frankly, failed quite miserably. It stung badly not only because of the words but because it came from a mature person of considerable talent, intellect, and potential. I felt responsible though Moses never hinted I was to blame. But I could not escape the fact that I had been a major part of his educational experience.

Moses had stood out from the other students, a sentiment apparently shared by the entire student body. They elected him president his first week on campus, a rarity given the multiracial mix of the people who unanimously voted him into the office. He did not disappoint their confidence. He was re-elected in his second year but then declined the next two years stating that other people should have the opportunity for leadership.

Moses had brought a steadying influence to our campus with mature thinking, dedicated scholarship, a disciplined work ethic—in addition to being humble, articulate, and honorable. All the things a faculty could hope for, especially a new faculty member like myself. Moses and I had connected well and could easily have been best friends were it not for the faculty-student protocol requiring formality and distance in such relationships.

Shuffling the curry and rice around on his plate, Moses continued answering my question. In summary, he said he did not feel that class material was connected to life issues he would be facing. Much of the lecture material, though well prepared and delivered competently, was never perceived as relevant. Little time was offered for class discussion. Students were left on their own to figure out how the material applied to their lives. He was told what to believe, what to memorize, but not how it connected to South African realities of apartheid. Being told *what* to think did not help him know *how* to think nor *how* to solve problems.[1]

Given the European influence in that region, the emphasis had been on taking good notes on the lecture material and passing the tests. In fact, faculty members were called "lecturers," indicating the didactic delivery of content. Thinking, reflecting, discussing, and applying truth seemed a remote part of the curriculum. It was assumed learners would make the transfer of knowledge into life on their own. Yet they had never been taught how to do that.

NOT MUCH BETTER

Other students from that time, Samuel, Sally, and Victor, had all shared their bumps in the ministry but somehow persevered and remained faithful to the Lord. In talking with these three former students I hoped the results might be better. They weren't. They mostly agreed with Moses, using more gracious words. But the meaning was the same.

They credited the teachers with being good role models. Taking weekend ministry assignments in local churches; being together for the weeklong practical ministry activities; laughing, praying, traveling, singing, and worshipping together—these were the things that seemed to help anchor these three lovely servants of God. The classes . . . not so much.

My confidence shaken, I began to wonder if I was really that bad a teacher. Of course, there were other faculty and maybe most of the blame could be shifted to them. But the conversations would not allow an escape. They did *not* include statements like "We are thankful, Mr. Elmer, that you were different from the others." My options were gone. I had to face my failure. Gathering the pieces of my shredded ego, I made a vow: I will dedicate my life to being a better teacher and helping others do the same. *Better* simply means helping people connect knowledge to life whether that knowledge be botany or the doctrine of salvation. In brief, I would like to be and help others to be informed practitioners, scholarly specialists, skillful professionals, insightful shepherds doing their jobs well while revealing the beauty of Jesus, "doers of the word, and not hearers only" (Jas 1:22 KJV).

Muriel and I have partnered these fifty years in this educational pursuit—her fields being curriculum, culture, health, and community development and mine being culture, communication, and educational processes. Both of us are trained in and committed to intellectual and biblical integrity in these fields. Thus, the birth of this book.

Both of us have been educators for all of our adult lives, in the home, in the local church, in educational institutions, non-formally, internationally, and domestically. Duane's first formal teaching came in South Africa in the early 1970s and for Muriel as a nursing instructor at a university in Michigan upon our return from Africa. Since then, both of us have taught at the bachelors, masters, and PhD levels. Muriel has focused more on culture, designing curriculum for community development and health care, much of it in the Majority World. Duane's education included curriculum and evaluation, human development, and cross-cultural communication. Both of us received our PhDs from Michigan State University at different times, and both of us have a formal Bible education.

Because our lives have been given to educational pursuits, it seemed natural we should coauthor the book drawing on the broad experience base now numbering nearly eighty years (combined) and in about a hundred countries. Readers please note that in the interest of easier reading, the use of "I" or "me" in chapters three through seven will refer to Duane unless otherwise noted. In chapters eight through thirteen, the primary voice will be Muriel's unless otherwise noted. In the remaining chapters we designate in the text.

We have found the words expressed by the apostle John—"I have no greater joy than this, to hear of my children walking in the truth" (3 Jn 4)—true. This is not to say that teaching is a utopia where only wonderful things happen. It surely is not that. And anyone in education for any length of time knows it. But we all know the effort is worth it. That being said, we are equally convinced that we can do better. That motivation to do better drives the purpose of this book.

WHO SHOULD READ THIS BOOK AND WHY

Our audience is composed of several groups, but our first audience is educators, especially those in higher education. This includes teachers/faculty, administrators, deans, provosts, and anyone involved in the education of students. Our deep commitment to the local church and the Christian school leads us to also include them as an important audience. Finally, we believe that anyone who teaches either formally or informally is educating. That would include parents, mentors, Sunday school teachers, coaches, consultants, disciplers, and anyone who tries to teach, nurture, or guide others. That's the *who*.

We can make this broad claim because we draw from the social sciences and neuroscience as well as the Scripture. The sciences have made enormous gains in recent years that help us better understand the teaching-learning process. We can benefit. That's the *why*.

SOME ASSUMPTIONS GUIDING THIS BOOK

While God reveals his truth in an absolute way, we perceive it dimly (1 Cor 13:12). The fall of humans into sin as a result of Adam and Eve eating the fruit in the garden of Eden has affected every aspect of life. Thus, while humans do not have absolute understanding of truth, our relative understanding is sufficient to believe in the Creator and to live God-honoring lives. This, of course, includes believing the trustworthiness of Scripture, the revelation of what the Creator has given to us including knowledge of the life, death, and resurrection of his Son, Jesus Christ. What we understand in part should not hinder any from trusting in the Maker of heaven and earth and living his truth to the best of our knowledge.

We also draw from the social sciences, the physical sciences (neuroscience in particular), and the humanities because we believe God reveals himself in these disciplines as well as others. With that in mind, we attempt a synergy of God's truth from Scripture and creation, that is, truth drawn from the sciences, humanities, and fine arts, all of which inform educational theory and process.

While much of our book assumes Christians teaching in the biblical sciences, we hope some of our illustrations using our Learning Cycle will alert those of you in other professions that the model works in a wide range of academic disciplines. Thus, we have used it with medical workers, community development people, nursing programs, culture sensitivity programs, entire faculties of smaller universities, conflict resolution conferences, multinational corporations, theological education conferences, as well Sunday school classes and even in pastoral roles.

God gives us his truth both from Scripture (special revelation) and from creation (general revelation); the latter, of course, includes truth from the sciences, humanities, and the arts. To this we add the doctrine of common grace, which for our purposes means that God has extended his kindness (grace) to all members of the human race.[2] In brief, this means that even those who are outside of God's salvation may discover and know God's truth from creation even though they neither acknowledge him nor thank him for it. In Isaiah we read,

> When a farmer plows for planting, does he plow continually? . . . [D]oes he
> not sow caraway and scatter cumin? Does he not plant wheat in its place,
> barley in its plot, and spelt in its field? His God instructs him and teaches him
> the right way. . . . Grain must be ground to make bread; so one does not go on
> threshing it forever. . . . All this also comes from the Lord Almighty, whose
> plan is wonderful, whose wisdom is magnificent. (Is 28:24-29)

Thus, we gratefully benefit from farmers, doctors, pilots, mechanics, and scientists because they seek truth from creation and share it with humanity.

We are committed to God's promise that as his children, we can depend on his Holy Spirit to show us his truth. As the Gospel of John reminds us, "But when he, the Spirit of truth, comes, he will guide you into all the truth" (Jn 16:13).

In addition to believing God gives us truth from Scripture and his creation and we depend upon the Holy Spirit for guidance, we make another assumption: the teaching profession can always improve. In "the teaching profession" we include all forms in which teaching and nurturing occur. Besides the classroom and more formal workshops, we believe activities such as mentoring, discipling, parenting, leading Bible studies, etc., could benefit from insights gleaned from the neurosciences and social sciences.

Parker Palmer offers this critique:

> The world of education as we know it is filled with broken paradoxes—and with lifeless results:
> • We separate head from heart. Result: minds that do not know how to feel and hearts that do not know how to think.
> • We separate facts from feelings. Result: bloodless facts that make the world distant and remote and ignorant emotions that reduce truth to how one feels today.
> • We separate theory from practice. Result: theories that have little to do with life and practice that is uninformed by understanding.
> • We separate teaching from learning. Result: teachers who talk but do not listen and students who listen but do not talk.[3]

To the extent Palmer is accurate, we intend for this book to address these and other concerns.

TEACHING FOR THE INTEGRATED LIFE: THE LEARNING CYCLE

For most of our teaching careers, both of us have extensively used the Learning Cycle described in this book in our classrooms, and it has informed all our curricular design decisions. It was built on a solid foundation of educational theory and research. The more recent research on how the brain learns has only reinforced the validity of our Learning Cycle and compelled us to write this book now.

Duane originally created this Learning Cycle as part of his doctoral research at Michigan State University in an attempt to reconcile major learning models of the day. These models tended to separate the *cognitive* (thought, reason, logic), *affective* (emotion and feelings), and *psychomotor* (behavior) aspects of learning as though they happened independently of each other rather than in dynamic interaction. All three aspects continuously overlap and play out together whenever we are learning something new. New information (or revisited information) enters our thinking (cognitive). The new information generates a positive emotion (affective) that might cause us to engage in thinking about it more deeply. Before long we can find ourselves thinking about what would happen if we tried to act upon that idea (psychomotor/behavior).

Academia, however, tended to focus primarily on the cognitive function *often to the exclusion* of the other two. Given a wholistic biblical perspective, Duane was concerned about integrating all three learning functions into a seamless whole so that educators would recognize that good learning requires all three aspects: cognition, emotions, and behavior. Sometime later, based on her research and experience, Muriel recognized the importance of naming and anticipating the barriers we encounter when we attempt to put truth into practice. What keeps us from practicing a behavior that we know is important? Teachers and learners do well to consider those barriers. So, we included barriers to good learning into the model. See chapters 8 and 9.

The reader will see the word *recall* at each level in the Learning Cycle model as well as in the text. Note that this is a specific directive to reflect on Scripture as the foundation and final reference point in our teaching. But content also refers to creation truth as well, so long as it does not contradict Scripture truth. So in Recall —"I remember the information" (Level I in our model), the content we commit to our minds must not be in conflict with what we know to be biblical teaching as best we can discern it. Thus, *recall* can refer to any content drawn from creation (e.g., physical sciences, humanities, etc.) or Scripture (the biblical sciences) with the view that Scripture is the final authority on topics it addresses.

RECALL
I remember the information

RECALL
with
APPRECIATION
I value the information

RECALL
with
HABIT
I do consistently

CHRISTLIKENESS
Character Integrity Wisdom

RECALL
with
PRACTICE
I begin changing my behavior

RECALL
with
SPECULATION
I ponder how to use the info

BARRIERS TO CHANGE

In Recall with Appreciation (Level II) we are reminded that values, feelings, and emotions are given by our Creator, but we reflect on our biblical moorings to guide us in their understanding and expression. If emotions become the authoritative reference point, our moorings are personalized rather than tethered in the truth of Scripture. Level III: Recall with Speculation deals with how to connect truth and life. How should truth guide us in our daily walk with God and in a troubled world? Life is filled with obstacles to the exercise of faith, a concern we deal with in the chapters on Barriers. Do we have a strategy to overcome the barriers we invariably encounter?

Following a realistic look at Barriers to Change, we begin the applied part of the model, Recall with Practice (Level IV). The beginnings of a new be-havior, a new obedience, often determines whether it becomes stable over time. What should we know for making a good start in a new practice that we believe will honor God? Recall with Habit (Level V) deals with the sus-tainability of obedience. Finally, our ultimate goal is Christlikeness—the overarching purpose for which we educate. This purpose is expressed in char-acteristics of *integrity*, *character*, and *wisdom*, a discussion of which forms the concluding chapter. We consider these three terms to be more represen-tative rather than exhaustive. Other similar words could be included. We also believe these to be worthy goals for any teacher, whether teaching in aca-demic or non-formal situations.

By observing the advertising, academic excellence along with leadership seem the dominant themes in most Christian academic institutions. Re-cently another theme is getting traction: service. One sees the collegiate in a work situation getting "down and dirty," helping somewhere in the world. While these are good benchmarks, shouldn't character, integrity, wisdom (spiritual formation) be the dominant themes? Sometimes a given de-partment adopts such themes but rarely the school. Why are we not seeing spiritual excel-lence as a priority for which we advertise the purpose of our educational endeavors?

> *Education is the most powerful weapon you can use to change the world.*
>
> NELSON MANDELA

The point is simple. Education is composed of knowing and doing, rhetoric and behavior, theory and practice, intellect and engagement, cognition and courage, orthodoxy (straight speaking) and orthopraxis (straight living), content and experience, knowing truth and doing truth. However it is stated, the end product is the same: the linking of life in the classroom to life in society. They must be seen as close friends, mutually informing and transforming the other.

Two Other Models

Taxonomies of learning have been around for some time. We mention two specifically. First, that developed by Krathwohl and Bloom, first published in the mid-1950s, has been widely used and updated.[4] This model provided the foundation for our Learning Cycle. Krathwohl and Bloom's three domains—cognitive, affective (emotion), and psychomotor (behavioral)—have been used extensively with enormous benefit. We see two limiting factors. First, the three domains are not integrated to represent the seamless nature of learning and living. Second, the cognitive domain, mostly valued in the academic environments, tended to stand alone as if it were the only important component for learning.[5] Thus, academia emphasized cognitive abilities to the near exclusion of affect and behavior.

As neuroscience has shown, however, *effective* cognitive function relies heavily on the *affective* (emotional) part of our humanness. In fact, affect (feelings or emotions) is now understood to be the *gatekeeper* for the cognitive functions of thought, reason, and logic. Neuroscience validates that we function simultaneously and somewhat interchangeably in all three domains. None of this was known when Duane created the Learning Cycle. However, when we became familiar with the more recent brain literature and insights from the social sciences, all converged to reinforce the value of the Learning Cycle. For analysis purposes we use "levels" to describe the Learning Cycle, which we will show to be dynamic and mutually reinforcing.

Another popular learning model is offered by David Kolb.[6] Kolb defines learning as the process whereby knowledge is created through the transformation of experience. He puts the individual's experience as the driving force for learning: an individual has a "Concrete Experience," followed by "Reflective Observation," then "Abstract Conceptualization," and finally "Active Experimentation." The four stages of his Experiential Learning Cycle have been revised since the mid-1980s. His work has found wide acceptance among educators, and we have been influenced by his insights as well.

In contrast, our Learning Cycle model attempts to put content (truth, facts) as the driving force for learning. While learning necessarily incorporates life experience including reflection, analysis, and revision, we are uncomfortable with experience being the fixed reference point. We laughed when a friend of ours who took his first trip to Africa announced that he was ready to write his book on Africa. But we all know people who use their experience to make pronouncements about the way things really are, much like the poem about the seven blind men and the elephant: each encountered a different part of the elephant but were convinced that the part they encountered was an accurate description the entire elephant. Experience may give partial truth or one's own truth.

For this reason, the first level, as stated above, is Recall—"I remember the information." Fact or truth is our starting point and the fixed reference point. It is not fixed in the absolute sense that new insights cannot be incorporated. We are speaking of fact or truth as best represented by our current understanding. Recall is repeated at each level simply because our Christian faith rests on content: the Scripture, the revelation of God. Thus, Scripture becomes the recurring reference point for knowing, feeling, and doing. The same holds for truth drawn from creation. Every discipline has its body of content from which it works. Variance exists among the teachers as to what they judge to be the content for their respective class, but usually some body of knowledge (content) is the reference point.[7] The Christian, working with creation content, must exercise greater discernment in determining what is true or factual.

BASIC NEUROLOGICAL FUNCTIONS

As you can tell from our educational backgrounds, we are anything but neurobiologists. Nevertheless, recent findings from neuroscience on how the brain learns offer intriguing suggestions for how we teach and how learners learn. We will only describe how the neurological system works where it is critical for understanding implications for teaching and learning. We will be referring to one of the more recent brain imaging technologies: the functional Magnetic Resonance Imaging (fMRI). With electrodes placed on various parts of the head, the fMRI allows neuroscientists to see how the brain functions during learning. David A. Sousa, one of the more prolific interpreters of neuroscience to the field of education, describes fMRIs this way:

> Any part of the brain that is thinking requires more oxygen, which is carried to the brain cells by hemoglobin. . . . [During the fMRI] the computer colors in the brain regions receiving more oxygenated blood and locates the activated brain region to within one centimeter (half inch).[8]

According to Sousa, neurons are the "functioning core of the brain." They carry electrical impulses along the neuro pathways (axons) to branch-like structures (dendrites), which then transmit the impulses across a space (synapse) via chemicals (neurotransmitters) to another neuron, and the process that will "either excite or inhibit . . . neighboring neurons" continues. "Learning occurs by changing the synapses so that the influence of one neuron on another also changes."[9] With about "100 billion neurons," the adult brain processes continuous data coming in from the senses, "to store decades of memories, faces, and places; to learn languages; and to combine information in a way that no other individual on this planet has ever thought of before. This is a remarkable achievement for just three pounds of soft tissue!"[10]

Neurons connect and change each other and develop "neural networks."[11] In Jensen's words, "cells that have fired together often enough to 'wire together'"[12] develop into neural networks. We will be using a few of these concepts but, for the most part, we have chosen to describe complex ideas using language for a wider audience, which will be easier to apply to our respective life situations.

CAUTIOUS SCHOLARSHIP

Writing a book about teaching and learning in light of what we now know about the brain represents a challenging, if not daunting, task. The brain research especially has been a rapidly growing and daily changing science. Our intention has been to utilize stable insights from the brain literature, avoiding the more speculative areas. This approach provides greater confidence for a sound foundation of knowledge and more confident application to teaching and learning activities. We believe these insights offer benefits to teachers, parents, pastors, mentors/coaches, disciplers—really, all who wish to intentionally nurture others—whose professions may not interact with such research much or at all.

Howard Gardner, Harvard University educator, warns of oversimplifying complexities and drawing unwarranted conclusions such as "The Brain works like X; therefore, you should teach like Y," or, "The Brain works like A,

and so students should learn in manner B." A few lines further he offers a
more reasoned approach:

> A range of sciences (and other disciplines) provide suggestions about how best
> to educate. None of them is definitive, but it would be foolish to ignore any of
> them, and we are best off if we try to draw on the range of perspectives, paying
> particular attention when the various indices point in the same direction.[13]

The "various indices" pointing "in the same direction" are what we hope
to capture. Our objective is to extrapolate the meaning of studies firmly
grounded in research from several disciplines—including theology—and
faithfully report them for the benefit of all who educate, formally or informally. Our intention is to extend the body of literature related to the broad
field of Christian education to the various forms of nurture in which we
engage in the church, the home, our Bible/book studies, youth ministries,
sermons, and even our personal quiet times with God. We aspire to offer
insights that make education more Christian. That is, we all can teach more
effectively toward our goal of obedience to the Scriptures and creation truth—
being doers of the truth.

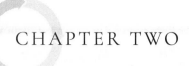

Weaving Truth and Life

Therefore, everyone who hears these words of mine and puts them into practice is like a wise man who a built his house on the rock.

JESUS, MATTHEW 7:24

Though there is no substitute for intelligence, it is not enough. There are human beings who have intelligence but do not have the moral courage to act on it. On the other hand, moral courage without intelligence is dangerous. It leads to fanaticism. Education should develop both intelligence and courage.

SIDNEY HOOK (AFTER FORTY-FIVE YEARS OF TEACHING)

E DUCATION THAT HONORS GOOD PRACTICE draws heavily from God's truth from creation. We hold that all truth is sourced in God and available to his people everywhere. As truth is examined, however, one must be more vigilant since much of creation truth is filtered through people not committed to a Christian worldview. That said, we all have filters; we "see through a glass, darkly" (1 Cor 13:12 KJV) and are prone to distortion. This alert should lead us not only to caution but also to humility in making claims.

With regard to truth, both of us owe much to the graduate faculty who taught us both at different times at Michigan State University (MSU).[1] We discovered that they were committed to discovering truth in their respective disciplines.[2] They showed us how to pursue truth and also to think about truth. Honest debate plus reading and listening to contrary opinion forged robust discipline of mind. Christian opinion and values were respected as much as anyone else's as long as they were delivered with a solid knowledge base and sound reasoning. Everyone's voice found a fair hearing. People felt safe. In that atmosphere we grew together in the discovery of educational theory and good practices regardless of our worldview.

Both of us had two small cohorts of like-minded people. They helped shape and guide the understanding and application of the material we had just explored together in the classroom and in the literature. One cohort community did not usually share our core worldview assumptions but extended respect generously to all by listening and engaging. The other cohort helped us think Christianly and encouraged the practices that were relevant to our respective worlds. We rehearsed the content we were getting, examined its values, and generally critiqued each other's thinking to guard against error or misdirection. Thus, as reflective practitioners we applied what we deemed important and determined its suitability for our work. This atmosphere of information and application energized us in ways previous educational experiences rarely did. While this did not happen all the time, it did with enough frequency that it frames nearly all our memories of MSU.

Little did we know that so many aspects of those positive learning experiences would turn out to be validated decades later by research on how the brain learns.

THE BEGINNINGS OF A MODEL

In the fall of 1974, following nearly four years of teaching in Durban, South Africa, Muriel and I returned stateside. I started a second master's degree at MSU while Muriel taught nursing at a local university.

Ted Ward, internationally experienced as an educational consultant and recipient of the prestigious Dag Hammarskjold Award (the only North American at that time to have received the award), would be my mentor—one of God's generous gifts to me. Little did I realize how my life and career would change from those years. Several years later Muriel was also privileged to have Ted Ward as her PhD mentor.

My master's degree rolled into a PhD program. Nearing the end of my doctoral studies, I was required to do what all the others had to do: comprehensive exams. There would be three questions, each written by me but modified or approved by my committee. At an appointed time, I would write for four hours on each question. One of those questions would prove exceptionally fruitful over the years. The question was this: *David R. Krathwohl and Benjamin Bloom created taxonomies for the cognitive, affective, and psychomotor (behavior) domains of learning. Explain each, how they might be conceived as an integral whole, and the possible effect on the vocation of teaching.*

While Krathwohl and Bloom wrote three separate books on the respective learning domains, as mentioned earlier, only the cognitive domain volume (authored by Bloom) really gained traction in the academic community. My goal was to see how the three domains could be forged as a more integrated model for understanding the teaching-learning environment. My answer to the comprehensive exam question emerged as five levels of learning best represented in a circular form.

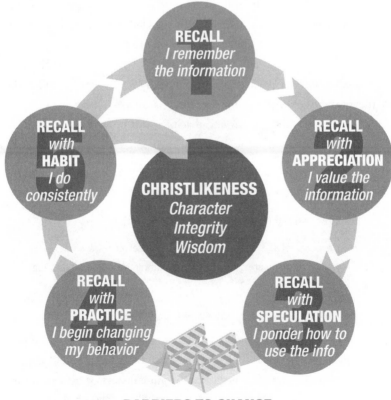

Levels I and II represent the cognitive and the affective domains respectively. But I felt there was a huge gap between those two and the psychomotor/behavioral (Level IV), application of truth to life. Here my doctoral studies in educational theory helped me fill in what I considered a void: the role of speculation (Level III) and the idea of continuity or habit (Level V)—a long obedience, sustained obedience, if you will. Muriel saw a gap I had missed and added "Barriers," a most necessary ingredient for being successful in weaving truth and life into becoming a whole person. Last, we realized "Habit" was not the goal but rather the last step on the way to building character, integrity, and embodiment of wisdom as the final goal. Thus, these are at the center of the Learning Cycle.

CHRISTIANITY'S MOST SERIOUS PROBLEM?

Years after the MSU experience, in reading Matthew 23, I realized that our proposed Learning Cycle, if faithfully taught, could help learners avoid the pitfall Jesus so furiously attacked in the religious leaders of his day. Let's think together about this because I believe it represents a major concern regarding theological education, Sunday school classes, sermons, and what has historically been called Christian education. You may want to read all of Matthew 23 at this point, but here are some excerpts that represent the text.

Jesus is talking to the crowds and disciples, but he specifically addresses the "teachers of the law and the Pharisees" (Mt 23:1-2).

So you must be careful to do everything they tell you. But do not do what they do, for they do not practice what they preach. (Mt 23:3)

Everything they do is done for people to see. (Mt 23:5)

They love to be greeted with respect in the marketplaces and to be called "Rabbi" by others. But you are not to be called "Rabbi," for you have one Teacher and you are all brothers. (Mt 23:7-8)

The greatest among you will be your servant. (Mt 23:11)

Woe to you, teachers of the law and Pharisees, you hypocrites! You shut the door of the kingdom of heaven in people's faces. . . . Woe to you, blind guides! . . . Blind fools! . . . You have neglected the more important matters of the law—justice, mercy and faithfulness. . . . You are like whitewashed tombs. . . . You snakes! You brood of vipers! (Mt 23:13, 16, 17, 23, 27, 33)

(These are selected portions to portray some of Jesus' claims against the teachers of the law and the Pharisees.)

Now consider this series of questions. Before you look at my answers (below), I suggest you answer for yourself and see if we agree.

1. During Jesus earthly ministry, against whom did Jesus level his greatest criticism?

2. Who were the Pharisees and teachers of the law?

3. Why was Jesus so critical of these religious leaders?

4. What is a hypocrite?

5. What makes hypocrisy so bad?
   (Take some time on this very important answer)

6. Why was Jesus so harsh, it would seem, toward the Pharisees' hypocrisy?

7. How did the Pharisees get this way?

Below are our answers. If you see it differently, that is fine.

1. My answer: The Pharisees and teachers of the law (Mt 23:2).[3]

2. My answer: The religious leaders.

3. My answer: They were hypocrites (Mt 23:13).

4. My answer: Someone who knows the truth but does not live according to that truth (Mt 23:3-10).

5. My answer: Because if there is a serious discrepancy between what we say and what we do, people will usually believe what we do. Actions speak louder than words! Our teaching may point people to Jesus, but our actions may point people away from him (Mt 23:13).

6. My answer: Their actions violated their own words, thus deceiving the people. The Pharisees were actually leading people away from the truth of Scripture rather than toward it. Jesus was harsh not out of uncontrolled anger or resentment but because they were denying that he, Jesus, was the divine representation of God. His perceived harshness was an attempt to shake them loose from their deeply held misconceptions. This shaking process is called *cognitive dissonance* or *disequilibrium* (more on that later). Change comes when a disruption of one's flawed or unbiblical beliefs lead to considering a better alternative.

Jesus was trying to get these religious leaders to see him as he really was: the Son of God and Savior of the world. Thus, this apparent harshness could actually be seen as an act of love. Jesus was trying to help them see truth so they could live truthful lives. Did the religious leaders change their opinion of Jesus? Did this tactic work? It would appear not (see Mt 26:57-68; 27:20-23, 41-43).

The last point needs mentioning: beliefs are the origin of our actions. But the beliefs must be grounded in Scripture such that they affect our character and integrity—thus, the words and acts being mutually reinforcing. The real beliefs of the Pharisees revealed themselves in their acts, suggesting the Scriptures they taught were never incorporated into their beings. Their habits revealed who they really were. Jesus was rightly indignant with their fraudulent lives.

7. My answer: I will let you answer this one on your own! But consider that they were the theologically trained, recognized leaders. Leaders, mind you! *Shocking*, is my reaction. What happened between the time they entered the seminary or Bible school of their day and this moment of severe reprimand? Our own answer is the reason for this book. Read on.

A GRIM REALITY

When we live truth, people see Jesus and the gospel more clearly. When words and deeds fail to mesh, the message is compromised, weakened.

One grim reality needs to be stated before moving on: yes, the Pharisees and teachers of the law got some harsh (but deserved?) treatment, but we all must recognize that the hypocrite resides within each of us—in me and in you. So before we point the finger elsewhere, we would do well to point it first at ourselves lest the hypocrite factor only increase.

It is easy to overlook our own hypocrisies. It is easy to tell others that prayer must be part of a disciple's lifestyle. But sometimes we

The term hypocrite *in classical Greek primarily refers to an actor such as one sees on the stage, but it came to refer also to anyone who practices deceit.*

DALLAS WILLARD, *THE DIVINE CONSPIRACY*

are struck by our lack of prayerlessness in the face of difficulties we face. It is easy to encourage parents to teach their children about God; but then we must ask, "Am I faithful in talking with my grandchildren about God?" It is easy to teach students how to facilitate discussion in a classroom, but then how often do we give in to time pressures and lecture the entire class period rather than posing good questions that stimulate thought and discussion?

In what ways am I (and are you) a hypocrite? Name it; confess it; let God remove it with truth in word and deed. Obedience, a long obedience, day in and day out, is never easy. But no other options are allowed for the follower of Christ, and for good reason: the path of obedience leads to wholeness and integrity surrounded by the riches of God's presence in this life and the next.

The Educators' Challenge and Goal

Now for the educational connection. Teachers desire students not only to know what has been taught in the classroom but also to live accordingly. Parents pray that their children grow up to live the principles taught in the home. Church leaders long to see parishioners' lives reveal the character of their Lord. Disciplers and mentors pursue congruency between knowledge and life decisions. Spiritual directors emphasize the outworking of spirituality.

One striking feature of Jesus was the absolute coherence of his teaching and his life. Truth spoken was truth lived. Words and life merged into an identical message, compelling for any open-minded person.

Parker Palmer's book *A Hidden Wholeness* describes this pattern of hypocrisy as "the divided life" and calls us to live the undivided life. The divided life, says Palmer, is a cancerous pathology eroding self and relationships. It is living a lie while deceiving virtually no one, at least not for long. Palmer continues:

> The divided life, at bottom, is not a failure of ethics. It is a failure of human wholeness. Doctors who are dismissive of patients, politicians who lie to the voters, executives who cheat retirees out of their savings, clerics who rob children of their well-being—these people, for the most part, do not lack ethical knowledge or convictions. They doubtless took courses on professional ethics and probably received top grades. They gave speeches and sermons on ethical issues and more than likely believed their own words. But they had a well-rehearsed habit of holding their own knowledge and beliefs at great remove from the living of their lives.[4]

David, in Psalm 86:11, longs for the same wholeness when he prayed, "Teach me your way, Lord, that I may rely on your faithfulness; give me an undivided heart, that I may fear your name."

Gandhi also saw the importance of an undivided life. When asked by a Western correspondent to summarize his message in one sentence, he responded, "My life is my message."

OTHER PERSPECTIVES ON THE CHALLENGE

Hypocrisy easily infiltrates people of faith leading to fractured lives, marriages, and homes. The effect on society is self-evident most especially in the fractured nature of our nation. *E Pluribus Unum* (from many one) ceases to exist except on our coins, or so it seems. The greater tragedy is that the various "tribes" or "identities" not only appear uncaring about the deterioration of oneness but seem to feed like piranhas on the brokenness. Divisiveness has grown into an art that ignores all ethical boundaries. If we live long enough with our fractured lives, does it become the new norm? Will hypocrisy overpower morality to the point it becomes the new morality? Does anybody want to live in that world? Christians must offer an antidote, not contribute to the problem. By what means can we raise up new generations of whole, godly, integral people whose lives become beacons of light for the love and grace of God?

Over forty years ago Larry Richards bemoaned the lack of transformed lives among Christians and offered his reason for this claim:

> We have attempted to change persons by contact at one point of the personality (the cognitive), and by the simple expedient of providing new (revealed) information. The result far too often has been the development of a distorted faith; a faith that takes the form of beliefs isolated from the total personality . . . divorced from body and emotion and divorced from doing.[5]

Distinguished sociologists like James Davison Hunter seriously question the possibility of morality returning to our nation. After dismissing platitudes-based behavior change (e.g., "Just say 'no'") he offers this foreboding prognosis.

> We say we want a renewal of character in our day but we don't really know what we ask for. To have a renewal of character is to have a renewal of a creedal order that constrains, limits, binds, obligates, and compels. This price is too high for us to pay. We want character but without unyielding conviction; we want

strong morality but without the emotional burden of guilt or shame; we want virtue but without particular moral justifications that invariably offend; we want good without having to name evil; we want decency without the authority to insist upon it; we want a moral community without any limitations to personal freedom. In short, we want what we cannot possibly have on the terms that we want it.[6]

We believe that Christians living lives of truth, integrity, and character can be agents of reconciliation that does not stop with the vertical reconciliation to God. It necessarily includes horizontal reconciliation to our brothers and sisters locally and globally. Teachers can make a difference toward this end.

We have been privileged to be teachers. We have loved the vocation. It has been our honor to know each person God has placed alongside us. But, as in any valued profession, there is a reckoning that we dare not ignore. The previous chapter explored Jesus' confrontation with the teachers of the law and Pharisees. That encounter strikes us as a caution, if not a warning, that teaching can be dangerous.

The Really Hard Question for Educators

Is it possible we unwittingly contribute to the hypocrite problem, the deterioration of character in our Bible schools, Christian colleges, seminaries, graduate schools, and church education programs (Jas 3:1)? Are we inadvertently graduating hypocrites by the way we elevate knowing truth (cognition) without corresponding emphasis on living truth?

We are raising the question because we must look at ourselves and attend to our own "world" individually and institutionally. In light of current knowledge are there adjustments we should consider that might help us do our jobs better? We would all like to think we are exempt from hypocrisy: *it is different in my classrooms.* We take rightful pride in remembering our graduates who became success stories. But what of those who failed? In this next chapter we will look more carefully at how we might do education better with the specific aim of nurturing the kinds of people who strive to live seamless, truthful lives revealing the character of Christ.

Recall

I remember the information

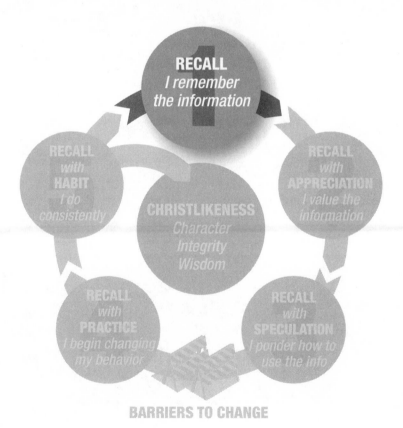

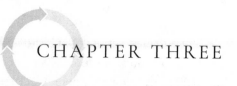

CHAPTER THREE

Recall, Rehearsal, and Retention

The memory should be specially taxed in youth, since it is then that it is strongest and most tenacious. But in choosing the things that should be committed to memory, the utmost care and forethought must be exercised; as lessons well learned in your youth are never forgotten.

ARTHUR SHOPENHAUER, 1788–1860

Reduce teaching to intellect, and it becomes a cold abstraction; reduce it to emotions and it becomes narcissistic; reduce it to the spiritual and it loses its anchor to the world.

PARKER PALMER, *THE COURAGE TO TEACH*

Then you will remember to obey all my commands and will be consecrated to your God.

NUMBERS 15:40

THIS CHAPTER STARTS WITH RECALL, the ability to remember. Without recall all our teaching is in vain . . . well, maybe not *all*, but much. While recall is the beginning, it is not the end. More than recall, teachers must promote deeper learning, which takes us into rehearsal and retention.

Picture the last sermon you heard. What was the topic? What Scripture was used to address the topic? Can you say what the conclusion was? How might that conclusion have made a difference in the hearers' lives? Were there things the preacher might have said to make the application more relevant to the hearers' lives? Often we cannot even remember for twenty-four hours the truth presented. Yet we are known as the "the people of the book." How can pastors and teachers enhance remembering so that they can get to promoting deeper, active learning?

LAUNCHING THE LEVELS OF LEARNING:
A MODEL FOR TEACHING AND LEARNING

Recall and remembering launches the model that eventually takes us to a point where truth and life are woven seamlessly to form character, integrity, wisdom, and godliness. But it starts with content. Teachers tend to think of knowing content as primarily a cognitive function. That is, we want facts to be known, to be registered in the brain and, as much as possible, to be committed to memory. But for content to be fully integrated, it must move beyond the memory function.

The task of the following chapters will be to chart this journey from remembering content to integrated learning that forms character and integrity. For now, we explore the essentials of knowing. We remind you that each chapter repeats "Recall" because remembering content is the foundation of learning. It is foundational because the teacher's goal is to help the learner ultimately arrive at the point where the content may no longer explicitly surface in the learners' memory as words but becomes integral to the life and character of the learner—a way of being. Truth, content, and information are terms used somewhat interchangeably in our text, a point noted earlier. When we reference Scripture, we more often use the term *truth* to indicate its authority.

THE BRAIN, MEMORY, AND LEARNING

Memory simply means the retention of information. How that retention happens and for how long has occupied neuroscientists for decades. In the last two decades the development of a sophisticated machine that shows actual brain activity has opened up new vistas of insights ranging from concussions, to learning music, to dementia, to virtually every area of life. Functional magnetic resonance imaging (fMRI) has exponentially expanded knowledge that assists in understanding, diagnosing, and treating various ailments as well as suggesting ways to improve conditions like education, nutrition, and aging.

Short-term memory, working memory, and long-term memory. There are three stages of memory: *short-term* (also called immediate or sensory memory), *working* memory, and *long-term* memory. Definitions and terms differ, but for this book we will use the following terms and definitions:

- *Short-term memory* refers to a very temporary storage of material often lasting only a few minutes up to a day unless something activates it to move into working memory; this is also called *immediate memory* in some literature.[1]

- *Working memory* refers to material that is being processed by the learner—for example, thinking about it, disagreeing, summarizing, discussing, debating, or applying.

- *Long-term memory* refers to material that has been acted upon by the person over time such that it enters into long-term storage in the brain available for use later;[2] the material is considered more permanent especially if the neural network continues to be strengthened by use; it is the place where basic assumptions, values, beliefs, and foundational truths about life are stored and from which behaviors emerge; only a change in the content of long-term memory will produce behavior change.[3] This is where religious beliefs are stored such as faith in God, the truth claims of Jesus Christ, authority of Scripture, etc.

Sometimes called *deep learning*, long-term memory is information that has been active in working memory to the point where it shifts into long term storage and, in the words of James Zull, becomes "learning that changes a life," the goal of education.[4]

Conditions Upon Which Learning Begins

Educational researcher David A. Sousa identifies two foundational conditions for long-term storage of information:[5] the material must make sense and it must have meaning (relevance), without which learning does not occur. If the material has both sense and meaning, the probability is greater that the material will move from immediate to working memory. With proper stimulation, the content may then move into long term memory, where it affects one's core beliefs about faith and life. More on this later.

Does it make sense? "Make sense" refers to comprehension; does the learner comprehend what is being said so that s/he can repeat it accurately in his/her own words? That which does not make sense is unlikely to be remembered. It is wise for the teacher to stop rather regularly and have someone summarize or review what has been said. This accomplishes two things, potentially: (a) it will determine whether learners are making sense of the material, and (b) your summary or a student summary may help others make better sense should any ambiguity exist. Make sure different people answer along the way, which will give you a good idea if the making sense is fairly widespread. Furthermore, it will alert you as a teacher where you may have been unclear.

Does it have meaning? Meaning refers to relevance, similar to "meaning making" or "meaning perspectives."[6] If the content stimulates the interest of the student or connects with content already stored in memory, or aids in decision making or helps solve a problem, it will have meaning. What teachers want to avoid is the thought all learners have at points: "What difference does any of this make?" Or, "I can't imagine how this will ever be useful to me."

An alert teacher might ask learners different questions at different times such as: "Why is this material important?" "Of what value might this material be to you?" "Who can give an illustration of how this content has been or will be useful?" A minute or two responding to questions could make a big difference. Plus, if you have been lecturing for fifteen minutes or so, students may be losing alertness and a question will bring them back.

Of the two—sense and meaning—meaning is a better predictor that the brain will make a connection with previously stored information. Each time a connection is made, that is, it both makes sense and is meaningful, the neural network related to the topic is strengthened. With further stimulation it may enter long term memory. "There is a neuronal network in our brain for everything we know," states Zull.[7] As these networks are strengthened through repetition, discussion, debate, reading, writing, rehearsal, and other learning tasks, the learning is made more permanent.

LEARNING AND RETENTION

The ability to recall information depends upon its being stored in such a way that it is available for use at a future time. Material memorized for a test is mostly stored in short-term memory and tends to be lost within a day or two of the test. One could hardly say the material has been learned, for it is lost so quickly and rarely affects any behavior.

Read the following. "Learning and retention are different. We can learn something for just a few minutes and then lose it forever."[8] Do you agree with Sousa's distinction? It sounds plausible until you think about your definition of learning. Oddly, Sousa never gives a clear definition of learning. But here we must respectfully disagree. To say something is *learned* if it has a life of a couple minutes or hours seems a stretch. By contrast, we believe something has been learned when it becomes part of the believing and behaving pattern of the person's life. To have learned is to have stored information in long-term memory where belief and behavior exist as a seamlessly woven part of the person's life. The five levels in our Learning Cycle represent the stages or "kinds" of learning that eventuate in a person having *learned.* Thus, *learning* is a progressive concept that incorporates cognition, affect, and early practice (living) the truth.

Rote memory and retention. Rote memory refers to the storage of facts that need to be recalled for specific occasions such as the times tables for calculating numbers or dates for delineating historical events.

To be sure students still learn their times tables, I (Duane) checked with my high school age granddaughter and she assured me that she had to learn (rote memory) her times tables in elementary school.

It is a legitimate form of learning and the retention can be critical to life itself. If you are in medicine, the names of bones or muscles are committed to memory. For the chemist, it would be the periodic table. For astronomy, other items will be memorized. For the pilot, the laws of aerodynamics. For me, it was the telephone numbers of my two uncles in the city where I attended college. They were my "lifeline" in this city where I knew no one and felt very vulnerable. Now fifty years later I can

> *Rote learning does not tend to facilitate transfer, but learning with understanding does.*
>
> DAVID A. SOUSA, *HOW THE BRAIN LEARNS*

recall them even though those numbers have been useless for the past forty years. But they stuck with me. For the Christian, important Bible verses and passages of Scripture, rote memory is useful.

For rote memory to function well it requires repetition. The repeating of certain data consolidates it in the mind through periodic or daily use or through disciplined review in order to keep the data fresh for retrieval. Not needing to "relearn" blocks of information allows the brain to use less energy in certain "automatic" tasks—to be more efficient—and frees it to attend to other priority functions.

Rehearsal and retention. If the educator—or anyone who provides instruction/nurture to someone else—wished for a magic "bullet," *rehearsal* would be a candidate. It might be hard to overestimate its value especially if accompanied by some other activities. And it is not really hard to do yet provides greater assurance that learning has been achieved. "There is almost no long-term retention of cognitive concepts without rehearsal."[9] *Rehearsal* is, simply, *meaningful* repetition, different from rote repetition in three ways:

1. Meaningful rehearsal involves repeating the information in one's own words but remains true to the original meaning. This skill reveals comprehension or understanding and indicates the learner has "made sense" of the content.

2. Meaningful rehearsal involves seeking personal application. For example, as I rehearse the fact that all people are made in the image of God, my mind asks, "What difference this belief should make in my thinking and in my relationships?"

3. Meaningful rehearsal involves promoting transferability. For example, connecting an idea with multiple contexts. In my workshops I sometimes talk about building trust with people who are culturally or ethnically different. A number of people tell me they found that concept helpful with their spouse or child. An idea in one context is extended into another context without distorting the original content. Rehearsal, the reflection on an idea, creates better data gathering, sharpens analytical skills, interprets situations more accurately, generates new possibilities, and proposes new solutions. This is often called "problem-solving."

Both Muriel and I have told our doctoral students that study at this level involves nurturing problem-solving skills. But those skills will glorify God only when they are exercised with humility so God is glorified and the church edified.

Rehearsal is necessary since learning is meant to affect core values and beliefs and, therefore, behavior. Anyone can do this. But it does take intentionality and discipline. You may have noticed already that some concepts have been repeated or we have suggested an activity the reader or teacher may wish to do. We have done this intentionally. There will be more repetition and rehearsal of certain material ahead—for the simple reason that these practices are necessary for the most important material to "stick," to enter working memory and hopefully long-term memory, where transformation happens.

Rehearsal is a powerful piece of the learning process that can occur anywhere: in class, in a textbook (electronic or paper), over a cup of coffee or tea, in an office, around the dinner table, through electronic media, in the pulpit—anywhere there is intentional retrieval of the information in order to intensify or deepen learning. For instance, each time we sing familiar hymns/spiritual songs filled with our beliefs, we rehearse what we believe (Col. 3:16). Those beliefs, reinforced once again, nudge us toward practice.

How Rehearsal Might Work: A Learning Task

Following is an illustration of the three points above regarding rehearsal. This relatively brief learning task helps move information into working memory.

As one step toward encouraging this deeper learning, we ask our students to write a "memo to myself," usually one-half to one page, in which they rehearse relevant content from the class time or the text or from conversation with someone else. We ask them to choose one meaningful thought or idea and express that in their own words. Then they are to write about why it has meaning for them and "to what end" or how this impacts their behavior.

Short and to the point, the memo to myself expresses something the learner has found valuable enough to write about and make part of working memory. The teacher reads it and responds. Getting the paper back, the learner reviews it, including our remarks (more rehearsal). The neural pathway is strengthened.

At the next class we ask everyone to share with a neighbor what they wrote; the listener comments on what they heard (rehearsal again).

> *You cannot recall information that your brain does not retain.*
>
> DAVID A. SOUSA,
> *HOW THE BRAIN LEARNS*

Each person gets two to three minutes to share and hear the response. The total time taken in class is only six to seven minutes, and now the neural pathway is even stronger and the content inches closer toward forming deep beliefs in long-term memory.

One might then ask each student to share their thoughts outside of class with another person, friend, spouse, child, or colleague . . . someone (re-hearsal again). In doing so the information further consolidates in the mind. Ownership of that material continues.

The degree of rehearsal noted above may seem "overkill." Maybe. But if the content is high value and core to building a strong worldview, then it will not be overkill but, in fact, the construction of a strong neural pathway that leads to and strengthens every fiber of truthful living.

Caution: too many memos to myself (or any task, for that matter) soon di-lutes the purpose of careful and continuing reflection on content. Thus, we do it at the end of a section or about every two weeks. However, at the end of a semester, for campus-based courses, we might ask them to bring all their memos for the final week at which time we ask each to select one or two (never more) that they want to commit to further reflection and application. We have found that more than one or two generally means none of them get ongoing attention.

My Own Experience

In my own experience, the doctrine of the imago Dei (image of God) may be among the most powerful doctrines for guiding relationships. Merely the *implications* were sometimes overwhelming. Realizing every human being carries the image of God means that every contact with another person either nudges them towards an "eternal splendor and glory or towards an eternal corruption and horror"[10] staggered my imagination. Paraphrasing C. S. Lewis, God intends for every human interaction to be a sacred moment. Any dehu-manizing of the person means we have profaned that moment and done damage to God's image in that person. The thought is stunning. Our worst profanity may not be cursing, bad as that is, but how we treat one another, including the stranger, the poor, the orphans, the widows, "the least of these."

Mitigating Circumstances

Among the privileges of teaching, perhaps the greatest has been the presence of international students in the classroom. Their presence represents the body of Christ from the nations. It also inspires confidence in the gospel and hope for the world.

Their presence in the classroom also presented challenges. Many students came from countries where the prominence of rote memorization did not en-courage independent thought. For others independent thought might even have been dangerous. They were superb at rote memory. Thus, giving back the same words they heard or read whether verbally in class or in writing for a final exam was not only expected but required for passing the class. Understanding was not valued as much as rote repetition even if meaning and clarity were obscure. Questions to the professor may have implied the professor did not do a good job of explaining and brought a reprimand rather than clarification.

That limiting factor created an additional problem for many international students in American classrooms. Rote memory was discouraged in their classrooms. So when American teachers called for comments reflecting understanding—that is, "express an idea or concept in your own words"—many international students had difficulty since neither thinking nor discussion were promoted in their home country. But the problem was compounded by their need to work in English, the second or perhaps third language in which they could function. Much of their education was memory for its own sake (and to pass tests, of course) but not discussion, debate, or the discovery of relevance.

Many faculty members fail to realize how much international students' past educational experiences had to be considered before evaluating the performance of these students, new to the Western classroom. For example, some confessed that they had been hit with a stick when they gave a wrong answer in class. Many recounted public humiliation and verbal abuse. Most admitted to fear as an ever-present emotion in their educational experience. Add to that the extra time and energy necessary to understand class content in another language and then to construct meaningful responses using alternative vocabulary to express understanding, one can only be amazed at their courage and discipline. Many spend long hours with English resources to perform their best. We should be humbled by their presence.

SUMMARY

Those of us who teach ought to do so in such a way that our content is clearly presented (makes sense) and has meaning (relevance) for the learner. This will be especially challenging for international students but with patience and understanding, they usually excel. Learning activities that cause learners to engage and rehearse the information will aid in assuring that information moves from immediate to working memory. The more that information is voiced, written, and applied, the greater the potential for it to enter long-term memory, where it becomes a deeply held belief and affects behaviors.

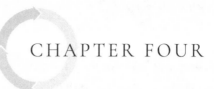

CHAPTER FOUR

Lectures that Transform

My son, do not forget my teaching,
but keep my commands in your heart.

<small>PROVERBS 3:1</small>

Repeat again what you hear; for by often hearing and saying the same
things, what you have learned comes complete into your memory.

<small>FROM THE *DIALEXEIS*</small>

R ECALL AND REMEMBERING, Level I of the model, eventually helps us see truth and life as woven seamlessly toward character, integrity, wisdom, and godliness. In this chapter we look at the reason for remembering followed by a perspective on the lecture, where it falls short, and how it can be useful.

ALTARS TO REMEMBRANCE

We will appreciate the value of remembering by first examining the danger of forgetting. Even a quick read of the Old Testament reveals a shocking memory loss for the Israelites. The following admonitions are framed in the context of warning and lament for having already forgotten:

- . . . be careful that you do not forget the Lord. (Deut 6:12)

- . . . Praise the LORD, O my soul, and forget not all his benefits. (Ps 103:2)

- ... do not forget my words or turn away from them. (Prov 4:5)

- ... [Who are you] that you should forget the LORD your Maker? (Is 51:13)

The consequences for forgetting God and his precepts are among the saddest passages in the Bible.[1]

As the Israelites traversed their land, they built altars of remembrance. The naming of the altars recalled an event in which God revealed himself in a special way. As families traveled, they would pass these altars, pause, and remember (rehearse). Those altar moments renewed memories of lessons learned and the call to be faithful to God (e.g., Gen 8:20; 12:7-8; 26:23-25; Ex 17:14-16; Josh 22:34).

Just as there were legitimate altars to remember the one true God and his acts, there were false altars erected by the heathen neighbors who worshiped idols—idols Israel was all too prone to adopt in spite of God's strict prohibition.[2]

Moses' words summarize what we are to remember:

> And now, O Israel, what does the LORD your God ask of you but to fear the LORD your God, to walk in obedience to him, to love him, to serve the LORD your God with all your heart and with all your soul, and to observe the LORD's commands and decrees that I am giving you today for your own good? (Deut 10:12-13)

Why the considerable emphasis on remembering in the Scripture? The obvious reason is that sin is forever present in this world and the temptation to wander from our Creator is always near and real. But the Creator may have had another reason for us to remember: the brain tends to function more efficiently and consistently when neural networks are stronger. For example, when one has a strong God consciousness—that is, reflects on God at various times during the day—that neural pathway becomes more dominant in our thoughts and actions. That pathway has "tentacles" (dendrites) that allow a wide range of experiences to connect to the God consciousness.[3] The more we connect life experiences to God, the good and the bad, the stronger our "altar" of worship and the more likely we will resist erecting false altars.

CONNECTING LIFE TO A GOD CONSCIOUSNESS

For example, while driving down the road you see an accident. You might realize that God has protected you and your loved ones and give thanks. But you might also realize that God is present with those in the accident and pray for their well-being, recovery, and—in the midst of all that entails—acknowledge him. Perhaps you might stop and be God's presence by helping.

But suppose you are the one in the accident. One tendency is to curse your "rotten luck," seethe in anger at the other driver, or curse the hassle of getting through this mess. A God consciousness interrupts those thoughts with, *God is here. He is present. What does he want to accomplish in this situation that I would have preferred to avoid? How then should I think and behave so that his presence will be apparent to the others who would also have preferred to avoid this misfortune?*

The strength of the God conscious neural pathway, from frequent daily use, creates a habit response that keeps God as the reference point for how we see and respond to life circumstances.[4] It goes without saying, no one is perfect. But it is also true that the formation of good habits will help us turn difficult times into "altars" of worship to our God. Those difficult life events can be cues that activate a thought habit, a God consciousness habit. We need to ask, *What do we want people (including ourselves) to remember about God after we walk away from a situation . . . especially the less than happy ones?*

MAKING THE CONNECTIONS (RELEVANCE)

The altars reminded Israel of their covenant God, and these reminders became connecting points for other life situations. In the same way, our learners, to make any sense out of content, need connection points to pre-existing content or experiences already imprinted in the brain—the "meaning" function. The brain waits to be stimulated with new material that connects with other content from past learning already stored there. This has been self-evident for decades among educators. Yet it seems not to have much traction in our classrooms as we jump into our lecture for the day assuming that the minds will immediately see the relevance to their lives. It is simply fallacious to assume learners will automatically "connect" to our lecture notes (or our sermons, for that matter).

Reuel Howe also comments on a common problem teachers' experience:

> Teachers and ministers seem to suffer widely from what I call "agenda anxiety" the anxiety to get across all the points of whatever subject they are dealing with regardless of the state of being of those whom they are teaching.[5]

The rush to get through is based on the questionable assumptions that:

1. The learners will return to their notes at some future date and "get it."

2. They will understand what they have written later.

3. The notes will prompt them to some relevant action later.

4. The learners cannot get the content anywhere else.

Think about these assumptions. How many are true of you? Did you review your class or sermon notes years later? And did they make sense? Did old notes prompt you to some behavior change? Or, when the need arose to review the same content, did you rather Google the material, read an article, or take a book on the topic out of the library rather than rely on your notes from class?

> *The major question is not how much material is covered but how much is learned.*
>
> DUANE ELMER

Doing less, better, is really a superior way. Failure to connect content with the learners' experiences, from the standpoint of transformation, is virtually a waste of time—or so the brain researchers suggest. Sousa says only what enters working memory may have a chance to enter long-term memory and affect core assumptions.[6] For the Christian, this relates to character formation and spiritual development.

Here's the point: teaching to pass tests, hurdle a barrier, hold up a piece of paper with embossed name and achievement, elevate oneself in a company, or build the retirement account miss the point. All of these are good, but they are not the goal of teaching and *should not* be the goal of learning. We teach and learn for wholeness; the undivided life; building the seamless tapestry of our character where our words and our actions merge as one, mutually reinforcing each other toward integrity—the journey to Christlikeness.

ENGAGING STUDENTS ILLUSTRATED

Here is my attempt to engage with my students' reality. In my undergrad cross-cultural ministry classes, I knew many of the students were there because the time frame fit their schedule or they were meeting a core requirement. Yes, some came quite motivated but still unsure if this class would be "worth it." My first words were: "This could be the best class you will ever take in preparation for . . . marriage," and when the amusement settled, I added, "because marriage is the biggest cross-cultural experience you will ever have." At that point, I had touched the hot topic that had been zip lining through the brains of these juniors and seniors since entering college if not well before. A palpable curiosity suddenly consumed the room. They learned that the skills for living in a new culture were parallel to those necessary for living with another person—even if they grew up across the street from each other.

When we teach, we are not simply teaching content, we are teaching people. People learn in certain ways that reflect the design of their Creator and that must be respected if our goal of maturity in Christ is to be realized. Teaching in a way that makes content memorable takes thought and effort.

THE LECTURE METHOD

Having observed and been involved in theological education in many countries, one reality stands out: faculty (and so many who teach in the home and church) still rely heavily on the lecture for content transfer. Doing so assumes that having delivered the "goods," the rest is up to the learners. This seems to be the underlying assumption in most classrooms. I think we have grossly overestimated what the learners do once they are exposed to the content. Their academic schedules, homework assignments, a job, possibly marriage, sometimes children, etc., rarely allow them time to do the proper reflection for material to go into short term memory much less working memory. Often, all they can muster is to get enough time to memorize the material to pass the next test.

Given that lecturing still dominates the delivery of content in most churches and theological schools, we will turn our attention to understanding it better with suggestions as to how the lecture can be more effective. Keep in mind that this material applies to all who teach in virtually any situation.

Assumptions underlying lecture.

1. Students learn best through lecture (telling).

2. Students are interested in the material.

3. Students will take good notes.

4. Lecturing facilitates retention of information.

5. Students will make their own applications to life.

Any of these assumptions can be true sometimes and for some students. I (Duane) for one, prefer more lecture while Muriel prefers more interaction. So we do not imply that lectures are wrong, but when examined, you may find they are weaker than you had hoped. That judgment will be yours, but we ask you make it at the conclusion of the book. Lectures can be made more effective, but it will necessitate less lecture time. In the end, though, we believe the results will be most rewarding. After all, if your lecture is packed with good content but they are not making any connections with what they already know or have experienced, it could easily be lost and your well-prepared lecture of minimal lasting value (at best).

THE BEST LECTURES

We have discovered that virtually everywhere teachers are committed to their students and desire most emphatically their mental and spiritual growth. We also assume that parents, pastors, disciplers, and Bible study leaders are no less committed. We salute that and join with you in that goal. That is also the goal of this book. As we learn more from the brain research and as data from student evaluations are considered, a growing consensus emerges about what good lectures look like.

We acknowledge that lecture is the default teaching style of many professors. We also acknowledge change can be daunting. Yet applying the insights we have experienced and now share has changed how we teach in nearly every situation. For example, we tend to use mini lectures of three to fifteen minutes followed by a learning task that requires the students to think and/or act on that content. We have found the rewards are worth the effort, very much so! Furthermore, we think you will not find it that difficult and, often, it is more engaging for everyone.

The best lectures build in learning tasks. Jane Vella's practical book *Taking Learning to Task* makes a strong case for open questions as one of the better "learning tasks." The common element in all learning tasks is that they engage the learners with the content.[7] She defined a learning task as "an open question put to learners who have all the resources they need to respond."[8] Neuroscience has overwhelmingly demonstrated that people learn best when the brain engages the content.

Hoffeld demonstrates how a question engages the brain:

What color is your house?

After reading that question, what were you thinking about? The obvious answer is the color of your house. Though this exercise may seem ordinary, it has profound implications. The question momentarily hijacked your thought process and focused it entirely on your house or apartment. You didn't consciously tell your brain to think about that; it just did so automatically.

Questions are powerful. Not only does hearing a question affect what our brains do in that instant, it can also shape our future behavior.[9]

One simple but effective learning task to engage learners is to ask a thought (open) question, which is likely to produce discussion versus the "correct" answer. Read these questions:

1. Do you tend to ask questions of your adult learners during class?

2. Would you be interested in learning how to ask better questions?

3. Is asking questions a good way to find out what people remember from the previous session?

4. When you lead a group, do you ask questions to find out what people are thinking? Their thoughts on a matter? Their experiences?

Now read this set of questions. What is the difference between this set of questions and the group above?

1. Why do you think a good teacher will plan to ask several questions during a class?

2. How does it make you feel when a teacher asks your group for your opinion on something?

3. What one thing should all teachers do to help the class get started discussing a topic?

(Possible answers include these: The first set required only short one-word answers. The second set called for more complete response including opinions, experiences or feelings.)

As you discovered, the first set were closed questions (also called convergent questions) designed to elicit yes/no or true/false single word answers or some specific fact. The short answer requires little depth of thought and closes off any further discussion.

The second set were open questions (also called divergent questions) designed to draw out the learners' assumptions, values, experience, and awareness as it relates to the topic. Open questions respect the independent thinking of the learners and tend to prompt discussion as students begin to compare their thoughts with the comments and opinions of others.

See if you can identify the open questions in this list and identify why they are open.

1. How many years have you been teaching psychology?

2. What is the difference between electrons and protons?

3. What are some skills a good facilitator should have?

4. How does the doctrine of the image of God affect your daily life?

5. Do you think chemistry is a difficult subject?

6. What are the various parts of a neuron?

7. How does Festinger define cognitive dissonance?

(Answer: The only two open questions are 3 and 4. Both 3 and 4 ask for an opinion. The rest of the questions are closed because they require yes/no or short right answers.)

Are there times when closed questions are acceptable? That, of course, was a closed question. It is a good idea to follow a closed question with an open one. In what circumstances might a closed question be acceptable? Adults will feel like they are being treated like children if you ask too many closed questions. Also, it will diminish their interest because the answers do not require thought. Rick Warren's discussion questions in *The Purpose Driven Life* are all thought-provoking, open questions.[10] Open questions tend to make people feel respected. Why do you think this is the case?

> *Questions hijack the brain. The moment you hear one, you literally cannot think of anything else. And that can be a powerful tool.*
>
> DAVID HOFFELD, "WANT TO KNOW WHAT YOUR BRAIN DOES WHEN IT HEARS A QUESTION?"

Teachers are very good at asking closed questions to elicit specific, correct answers. Creating open questions may be difficult at first. Practice turning each of those closed questions (above) into open, thought questions. Remember my questions (chapter 1) regarding the Pharisees and the teachers of the law: most were open; a few were closed.

For greater impact, Muriel always includes her open questions in her class notes, prepared ahead of time. Open questions posed to learners serve various purposes. Here are just a few: ask how the content relates to their experience (relevancy), ask them to identify content that is important to them and ask why (values), ask them how they might use the content (behavior), ask what outcomes they might expect when they put the content into practice or ask them what would keep them from using the content (barriers to change). Given some thought, you can come up with many more. Some teachers make a practice of taking Bloom's taxonomy of cognitive thought, mentioned earlier, and craft questions to meet those criteria. Although a good start, remember that the taxonomy only deals with the cognitive, Recall level.

Remember the "memo to myself" suggested in the previous chapter? Essentially it is a learning task with extended open questions, a one-pager. Respond in writing to three open questions:

1. Choose an idea from class that you consider to be important (the resource being the class or class reading).

2. Why is that idea important to remember?

3. Describe how that idea might prompt a need for change.

For less formal contexts, such as a Bible study group, the same learning task sequence may be used verbally. Ask the learners to think about something they considered important from the study and why that is important to them. Then ask them to share that with the person sitting next to them. If the group is small enough you could ask that they share it with the group. Then ask another open question: "What difference could this idea make in how you live your life this week?" And, ask them to share that with a neighbor or the group.

If you primarily lecture, it is possible your learners will have some difficulty with open questions early on. They may think you are looking for the "right" answer. When that is not obvious, they remain silent. Do not despair if they are slow to respond. They need time to think. "Thought questions" should be followed by a pause. You might start by having them give their response to a neighbor next to them so that everyone is engaged. When they are comfortable, they are more likely to speak openly in class. This learning task need not take much time but serves some valuable purposes. The regular incorporation of open, thought questions

- inspires positive attitudes.
- increases comprehension.
- develops ownership of content.
- increases motivation to follow through on application.
- increases attention to lecture material.

The best lectures honor retention times.

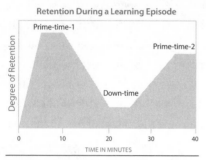 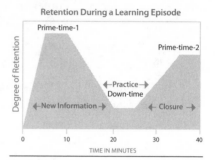

Figure 4.1. The degree of retention varies during a learning episode. We remember best that which comes first (prime-time-1) and last (prime-time-2). We remember least that which comes just past the middle.

Figure 4.2. New information should be presented in prime-time-1 and closure in prime-time-2. Practice is appropriate for the down-time segment.

The graphic above represents the way a typical brain functions during a forty-minute lecture. Neuroscientists, using an fMRI, tracked the amount of activity in the prefrontal lobe, part of the brain having to do with thinking, reasoning, and logic. White dots on a computer screen signaling activity registered highest during the first ten to twelve minutes of a learning session (prime-time-1) then dropped rather quickly. Around the seventeen to eighteen–minute mark the typical brain enters a "rest time" also called a *downtime* for approximately twelve minutes before increasing in activity for the balance of the session (prime-time-2). Keep in mind, the learner may still take notes and even show attention during the downtime. But reasoning or thinking fall well short of optimum.

Several parts of this figure are important for adjusting one's lectures to be more compatible with the attention rhythms of learners—and to keep the brain engaged!

1. Lectures should start almost immediately since that is the point at which the mind is most ready for information. Leave class attendance,

announcements, and extraneous material until the very end, when
most learners have already shut down even though the computers may
still be open.

2. The first part of the lecture should not be longer than fifteen to seventeen minutes because by then most students will have "tuned" you
out in favor of almost any other thought activity.

3. Somewhere in that fifteen to seventeen–minute window, change your
pace. Do something different. This can be an open-ended question, an
illustration, a personal experience; let the students talk one-on-one for
a minute each on summarizing what the lecture has been so far, or
what was most important, or what seemed most relevant—anything
that will re-engage their prefrontal cortex (in my lay language, their
"thinking apparatus"). Sousa calls this "practice" though I would prefer
engagement. Even a rhetorical question with a pause or an illustration
often works to "restart" their thinking allowing you to continue with
some assurance that the learners are with you again.

Many people enjoy TED talks. Have you noticed most are relatively brief—
around eighteen minutes? Do they hold your attention? Do you feel like it
was a learning experience? Did you think about it later? Discuss it with
someone else? Did it cause you to reconsider some aspect of your thinking
or behavior?

Further analysis of the TED talks reveals that they usually stay on one
theme or topic. They deal with that topic from several angles. Illustrations,
slides, and video clips highlight the words. Frequently one senses the emotional element in both the speaker and within oneself (see next chapter). The
presentation makes sense—that is, it is easy to understand—and it has relevance or meaning for the audience.

Prime-time-2 may contain additional lecture but should also allow for
further and more extended learner engagement. Since most class periods are
fifty minutes long, the astute lecturer will plan for two "practice" or "engage"
times, each spaced about fifteen to seventeen minutes apart.[11]

David Goodman notes: "Whether preaching, teaching, or leading a Bible
study, forget about holding their attention; think in terms of regaining their
attention. Our minds are too active for any communicator to hold us firmly
in their grasp for very long."[12]

The Beirut lecturer. At a theological educators' conference in Beirut, Lebanon, I was listening to a professor lecture for seventy-five minutes, a deadly length of time to hold anyone's attention. Yet I was surprised to find myself listening attentively in spite of the topic being rather remote to my interest. I confess my mind drifted to an analysis of this rather unusual circumstance (yes, that would be downtime, and I confess there were several). My analysis revealed rather enlightening data. The person, with mostly a monotone voice, would ask an open question about every ten to fifteen minutes. The question became a reflection on what had just been covered as well as a transition to the next body of material. Ingenious, I thought. If you choose to lecture, do it in a way that honors the listeners' attention spans. Rare is the person who can hold anyone's attention for seventy-five minutes. Looking around the room, however, not many of the fifty or so listeners showed they were attentive, suggesting his rhetorical questions had little effect beyond a few of us. So what can be done?

Sousa argues prime-time-2 should include time for closure when students consolidate the content by working on comprehension and meaning-making—does it make sense, and what does it mean? In the words we used earlier, prime-time-2 can be a time for rehearsal—does it make sense, and can I repeat the idea in my own words?—and reflection, a time for identifying personal implications regarding behavior change (meaning making) and then setting goals to that end. Prime-time-2 should include sharing with others the results of your thinking.

When sharing your thoughts, the brain becomes more active, and the content being thought about goes from immediate to working memory, where stronger neural networks are being constructed. If this content is rehearsed again by telling someone else, the neural network is further strengthened. If the brain continues to focus on the content over time, the content settles into long-term memory, where it affects values and beliefs, as previously stated. This process works for any content, good or bad, true or false. One immediately realizes the value of rehearsal for biblical knowledge. For that content to have any effect on building character and a life of integrity, it needs a process that encourages long-term memory. Note that rehearsal is critical to strengthening a neural pathway be it physics, literature, or biology.

Jensen comments,

> Either you can have the learners' attention *or* they can be meaning making, but
> never both at the same time. Meaning is generated internally, and it takes time.
> External input (more content) conflicts with the processing of prior content
> and thoughtful reflection.[13]

Jensen is saying, contrary to popular opinion, that the brain does *not* multi-task. Either it is processing content or it is creating meaning from that content. If the teacher keeps piling on content, there will be no space for the meaning of the content to enter one's own thoughts, and thus the "personalizing" of the material (making sense and meaning for oneself) will be lost.

Because comprehension and meaning making are not concepts most of us have been taught, it is unlikely that it will happen outside of class and unlikely it will happen in class unless the teacher is intentional about it—but it *should* happen since behavioral change depends upon it. One effective way to make it happen is by providing space for rehearsal during class.

The best lectures respect and compensate for downtimes. Most of us conduct our lecture as though every minute is the same. It is just not true. After fifteen to seventeen minutes into a forty to fifty–minute lecture (prime-time-1), the learner experiences a downtime of about ten minutes. During this time a part of the prefrontal cortex of the brain shows little activity on the fMRI, suggesting reason, logic, and thought have slowed or ceased. These time frames depend, to some extent, upon the students' level of interest and other factors.

We can bring them "back" into the flow of our material with a brief learning task. An illustration always attracts the attention of most; an open question nearly always alerts everyone. A brief activity abbreviates that downtime and rekindles interest in the topic. We suggest a two-minute learning task such as, "Turn to your neighbor and share an important insight or truth from the topic covered so far. You each get one minute." Note that while some will be eager to do this, others will be a bit hesitant (introverts?). Our experience suggests that the more introvert types (or the international student) may be given a "pass" for one reason: early on some may be a bit uncomfortable sharing but eventually all willingly engage. Our experience would verify this. It's permissible for some not to engage and not to try to force them. Let it happen in its own time. Then they will experience the joy and learning power of such activity rather than the awkwardness or fear.

Activating their minds will inspire their continued attention. Such a brief activity recalls important information in the mind of the learner, positions it in working memory because they had to construct their thoughts—at which point the element of ownership enters. Generally, even such a short activity not only stops the slide toward downtime but brings people "back" with a better attitude and higher level of interest.

Please consider using a major chunk of prime-time-2 (the second half of your lecture) for closure. Almost certainly it will reap the benefits of clarity, priority of content for each individual thought, and expression of an important insight. These learning tasks will activate the brain and move relevant information from immediate into working memory, where the Holy Spirit can eventually use it to bring about God-honoring change.

The best lectures are sprinkled with illustrations, passion, and surprise. One of the most popular—and I would also say effective—teachers in my department lectured much, but not all of the time. Students flocked to his classes, raved about his classes and were genuinely inspired to live for Christ as a result. His "office hours" sheet was filled weeks in advance. His classes were the first to be full and usually had students sitting on the floor because he allowed an overflow in registration. I watched him for several years. He delivered good content. His illustrations were often humorous, sometimes dramatic, and always drove home the teaching point.

It should be noted, too, that he knew everyone by name and something of particular interest about each. After class, in the halls, on the grassy areas, in the dining hall, he could be seen talking at length and, frequently, bowed in prayer with his hand on the shoulder of a student. Is it any wonder he was so loved and his influence profound?

He also used voice modulation that simply captivated. He paced, his arms flailed, he would turn suddenly silent; then, with voice low and serious, state why this was important to everyone in the room. Students hung there waiting for him to finish the sentence. He was not acting; he was genuinely passionate. Then, he would straighten up, survey the jammed room, every eye fixed forward, and out of the blue, fire a question: "Sister so-and-so, do you agree with what I just said?" Or, "Brother so-and-so, what would you have done had you been there?"

Sometimes he asked them straight-out content questions based on the assigned reading. I marveled at the respect they had for him and for the respect he showed them. Now, years removed, many will still say his was among the best classes in their four years on campus. Lectures are not bad, but they can be poorly delivered when they don't take into account good learning principles. And, truth be told, not many of us can lecture the way this professor did nor should we try. But there are insights and adjustments we can adopt to improve our own style.

As important as your presentation is, of equal value is the likelihood that if your enthusiasm, illustrations, discussion questions, and surprises spark their interest they will likely imitate you in their teaching—and preaching. Haven't we all done or tried to do some imitation of people who made learning come alive for us? Not only do we teach content, but we also show how to teach it (or, sadly, we may show how *not* to teach!).

Parker Palmer, having asked students the traits of their favorite teacher, discovered one stood out: passion, or enthusiasm. By contrast, he says:

> Bad teachers distance themselves from the subject they are teaching—and in the process, from their students. Good teachers join self, and subject and students in the fabric of life.
>
> Good teachers possess a capacity for connectedness. They are able to weave a complex web of connections among themselves, their subjects and their students so that the students can learn to weave a world for themselves. The methods used by these weavers vary widely: lectures, Socratic dialogues, laboratory experiments, collaborative problem solving, creative chaos. The connections made by good teachers are held not in their methods but in their hearts— meaning heart in its ancient sense where intellect and emotion and spirit and will converge in the human self.[14]

Over the years I (Duane) have taken informal polls asking the question: "What contributes to good learning in the classroom?" The following five answers emerged (not in any rank order):

- Teacher has a passion for the subject.
- Teacher connects the material to the students' reality.
- Teacher engages the students in the learning process.
- Teacher has a positive perception of the student.
- Teacher knows the material well.

But what of the quiet teacher, one who is not much for showmanship or voice modulation or adventurous stories who just teaches (or preaches) in a way consistent with who they are? All types must be respected, for everyone called by God to a vocation has something to offer. But not one of us teaches perfectly, so let's learn from one another.

Recently a special speaker, a quieter type, came to our church. At first I wondered if he would hold the attention of the rather large congregation. But soon his exquisite vocabulary, sentence construction, illustrations, humor, and astounding insight into the Scripture (a rather remote Old Testament passage at that!) transfixed us for the next forty minutes. We worshiped, felt God touch our conscience, and resolved not to live in resentment but to forgive, to trust the sovereign God who calls us to live in the freedom of forgiveness because he has first forgiven us.

We can be true to ourselves in the classrooms and the pulpit and in the home. Yes, learn from others because none of us does it perfectly. But then work hard to make it interesting, relevant, and practical. But always use some classroom time for students to engage with each other and the content.

The best lectures slot in reflection times. Consider another dilemma educators face: "As faculty with too much to cover, we sometimes do not spend the necessary time to find the aspect of our subject that will excite our students and then we complain when students are disengaged."[15]

When we fall behind in our notes and begin to rush, students may still take notes, but it is mostly mechanical. Students are unlikely to "get it" at some future date. Besides, they can get the content through multiple sources in today's electronic-rich world. What they need is someone to help them reflect on the content, some aspect important to them, and create meaning for their life and ministry. Without reflection time, content tends to remain impotent.

Learning tasks for reflection. Whether in a high school or college classroom, Sunday School class or Bible study, I would take about fifteen to twenty minutes at the end of a major section, series of sermons, or end of semester and ask everyone to answer the following questions (i.e., engage in a learning task):

1. Look over your notes and select something important to remember that should affect your life. (This gets at Level I: Recall and Level II: Recall with Appreciation.)

2. What specifically will you need to do differently if you are going to follow through on this change or these changes? (This gets at Level III: Recall with Speculation or, "What might I do?")

3. List hindrances or barriers you may encounter when making these changes. (The chapter on Barriers is ahead.)

4. Who will you want to join you in prayer and to journey with you as you follow the Lord in this decision? (This is Level IV: Recall with Practice.)

5. By God's grace you will be successful in this venture. Assuming so, who will be affected, including yourself? (This is Level V: Recall with Habit.)

Most people are astonished at how many others will be positively affected when they strengthen their own walk with God. But ultimately even God is affected by our obedience. The Old Testament book of Leviticus is filled with the obedience offerings of the Israelites and the statement that they were an "aroma pleasing to the Lord." In Revelation the prayers of the saints are a sweet incense in the nostrils of God (Rev 5:8; 8:4). God finds pleasure in our obedience! We can prompt obedience in our classes and sermons.

In helping people take time to reflect, we help them establish a lifelong habit they can use not only with themselves but whenever they nurture others. One must not do it too often or it can get tedious. But do it we must. Both the thinking and reasoning parts of our brains are activated as well as the emotional part, as we shall see ahead.

It is not a good idea for anyone to make a very long list of items they want to change. It almost guarantees they won't do any of them. The list gets overwhelming and either procrastination or paralysis or both settle in. Better for your students to make one (at the most two) meaningful changes as a result of a given course or series of Bible studies or Sunday school classes or sermons. Better just one action done well than lots of good intentions and no change at all!

The best lectures create meaningful conclusions. Most educators believe *closure* (i.e., bringing a class, study, speech, or sermon to a meaningful ending) should be intentional at the end of most classes. These are usually much briefer than reflection times but serve the purpose of consolidating what was important. Here are some ways to end a session: a summary by a teacher (or even better, by a student), an application, an insight, a new idea, a point of debate, a meaningful thought—even an open-ended question, a quotation, or something Jesus did.

One of the best educators I ever knew was also a colleague in another department. His style was closer to mini-lectures, seven to ten minutes or so, and then dialogue. His classes were also well attended. He closed every class with two to three minutes of some kind of student summary statements usually taking various forms I just noted.

Miscellaneous merits of lecture. A lecture can:

1. *initiate interest* in a topic especially with questions that link content with something relevant in the lives of learners if done with enthusiasm.

2. *pose a problem* (as in problem-based learning) for which a following activity will provide resolution or resolutions.

3. *provide necessary knowledge* for the class to perform some function.

4. *summarize*, especially if time does not permit student engagement to do so.

5. *express one's own opinion* or *provide illustration* of some concept.

6. *expand on a point* brought up in class but not accessible otherwise.

We already noted that we are not strong proponents of fifty to sixty–minute lectures. Thirty minutes might be a stretch unless some of the strategies provided above are utilized. We are strong proponents of mini-lectures or lecturettes that effectively accomplish some of the items immediately above, and others available in the literature.[16]

LIMITATIONS OF RELYING ON LECTURES ALONE

While some lectures can be motivational, it depends heavily on the lecturer. Many of us are stricken with less-than-ideal presentation skills. For the majority of us, it would seem, we must be aware of some limiting factors when relying heavily or exclusively on lecture.

Cognitive load. Cognitive load, also called "cognitive capacity" refers to the amount of time and volume of content a given person can meaningfully process before mental fatigue sets in.[17] Earlier we noted optimal retention times (prime-time-1 and 2) each lasting about fifteen to eighteen minutes with a down time of about ten minutes between them. The brain functions at optimum levels during the opening minutes of any teaching session. As one approaches the fifteen-minute mark or so (it differs according to individuals), brain processing seems to slow unless some intervention resets it for renewed attention. Thus, we must think of a sliding scale of higher or lower cognitive processing depending upon various individual factors, with time being the important one.

Another group of researchers note that "*germane*" material, that is, material the learner perceives as highly relevant, allows for greater cognitive capacity than does extraneous material.[18] In fact, "Whereas extraneous cognitive load interferes with learning, germane cognitive load enhances learning."[19] In other words, the learner has less cognitive capacity for processing material perceived as irrelevant or disconnected from life, and whatever learning may occur is poor. By contrast, relevant material is processed more deeply and produces quality learning.

Cognitive overload. Cognitive overload, also called "cognitive fatigue," means that people can "max out" on information.[20] They reach a point where rational thought shuts down. People may proclaim they are "brain dead." Most have experienced it when taking back-to-back classes or attending nonstop meetings at a conference.

When the mind has been bombarded with information continuously—morning, afternoon, and evening without proper rest intervals—decreasing cognitive activity registers on the fMRI. Different people reach overload at different points. But each experiences the same result: at some point the brain stops processing, the listening ceases, the mind wanders, words keep coming but nothing sticks. Sousa notes further that for adolescents and adults, "cognitive fatigue" sets in after ten to twenty minutes depending upon the individual.[21] This is consistent with the fifteen to eighteen–minute intervals in which people are most attentive. It does not matter if the material is interesting; it is still too much. People may appear to be paying attention, but a closer look reveals a glaze in their eyes. Bonwell and Eison report this happens even with medical students, where one assumes high motivation.[22]

So what do you do if you are the fifth or eighth speaker right before the evening meal? (Or if your session is the last class of the day?) It's an unenviable place to be sure. Here are some suggestions. Since the brain craves activity, get them active for a minute or two. Have them stand and share with someone near the best thing they experienced that day. That simple task activates their mind, allows them a moment of reflection and consolidation. Finally, it gives them a chance to talk. They will be revived and alert for when you begin teaching. Then keep your presentation short. They will almost certainly remember you favorably. It has never been easy to sit and listen for fifty to sixty minutes but even more so in the age of electronics, when images change on the screen every few seconds.

But the lecturer must be careful or an even worse malady awaits.

Cognitive unload. Surprisingly, people just don't walk away when they get saturated with content, they may "unload" it. If they are required to keep attending more content sessions, their attitude turns negative and not only do they stop processing, but they now lose whatever benefit they derived from earlier sessions. Their emotions turn sour, learning ceases and, may, in fact, reverse, losing any previous learning gains.[23] The next chapter on emotions will explain this further.

Many of us have had physical experiences that are similar. The food is good, you eat lots, you keep on eating and feel full; but still, you eat just a little more until you realize that unpleasant feeling in the stomach signals that you have overdone it. That which was so good has become distasteful—and maybe worse!

My experience suggests that many Christian conferences (and Christian schools), in the desire to get as much "good food" into peoples' heads as time allows, simply overdo it, and the good is lost. It's all good content, but it's still too much good for good learning.

I have similar memories from my earlier years of sixty to seventy-minute sermons, elongated family devotions, and youth meetings that can best be described as "sit and listen."

An educational proverb applies here: "When you get numb on one end you get dumb on the other."

REFLECTION POINTS FOR LECTURERS

The limitations below represent reflection points for those of us who teach in more formal settings. By noting these limitations, we may be able to "fix" them or, at a minimum, mute their negative effect on learning.

1. The lecture is not a good use of class time, especially if the material is available elsewhere.

2. Students tend to get bored, another way of saying the brain is not engaged.

3. Getting an "A" in the class is a better indicator of good memory than having learned.

4. Mindless note taking rarely gets beyond short term memory and rarely into working memory; content in short term memory disappears in one to two days unless stimulated by rehearsal.

5. Lectures alone tend not to affect behaviors.

6. Lectures tend not to produce higher order critical thinking skills.

7. Lectures tend not to change attitudes.

8. Lectures tend not to create transferable skills, necessary in a complex world.[24]

People who lecture should not be discouraged by these comments unless you lecture exclusively. In that case, you should consider your student and peer evaluations; also consider whether or not your students are meaningfully engaging the material, "owning" the knowledge, and being empowered for life in new and/or better ways.

SUMMARY

Lectures were required in earlier times when books were not available and lecture was the only way people could acquire information. While lecture should not be relegated to antiquity, we must recognize there are many more ways to access the information and, in many cases, these ways are superior. Experts (teachers) remain valuable, necessary, and strategic but will be more successful if they add additional skill sets to their lecturing. We have tried to respect the lecture mode especially if considerations from the brain research are incorporated. Then they can be a useful means by which people learn in all the good ways we noted above—and more good ways ahead. Read on.

Recall with Appreciation

I value the information

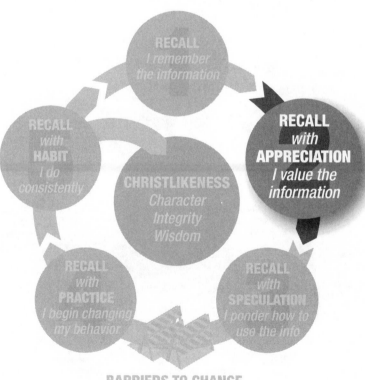

CHAPTER FIVE

The Role of Emotion in Learning

Above all else, guard your heart, for everything you do flows from it.

PROVERBS 4:23

Education without values, as useful as it is, seems
rather to make man a more clever devil.

C. S. LEWIS, *THE ABOLITION OF MAN*

Without emotion, learning is impaired.

M. IMMORDINO-YANG AND M. FAETH, *MIND, BRAIN, AND EDUCATION*

Emotions consistently affect attention and learning.

DAVID A. SOUSA, *HOW THE BRAIN LEARNS*

*A*T AN IMPRESSIONABLE AGE of about fourteen, I became strangely enamored with golf—strangely, because it was some distance to the nearest golf course for this country kid. I was too young to drive. My father could see no purpose in the game and therefore did not support my interest. One Wednesday night prayer meeting I sat next to an elder in the church, a single man about my father's age and among the most kind, gentle, and sensitive men I knew. He drove a huge eighteen-wheeler semi, which made him a superman in my estimation. He asked how things were going. I made an offhanded remark about wanting to play golf someday. He chuckled and said, "I play a little golf. Would you like to go with me some time? I could teach you the little I know." Wow, I jumped on that invitation but countered with, "I don't have any clubs." He quickly responded, "That's no problem, we can rent some."

I had never been in a golf clubhouse or even walked on a golf course, so this was all new. We played a few Saturdays later. He paid all my expenses. As I made a bunch of horrible shots, he would make only affirming remarks: you have a good swing; try standing a bit closer to the ball; for your first time you are doing well, and so it went. I played a horrible game, but why did I feel good? It was a day of uninterrupted affirmation, encouragement, and gentle help.

He quickly realized that I enjoyed the game and after our third outing he said: "My boss wants me to work more Saturdays, so I will not be able to play any more this year. Why don't you take my golf clubs, my gift to you, and you can practice around home. Maybe someone else can take you to the golf club. I would love to continue but it's not possible at this time."

The story may appear to be a kind gesture on the part of a generous man, but it was far more to me. Here was someone who said, in essence, "You are important, important enough that I will give you several Saturdays, my golf clubs, and my interest."

"I value the relationship. I want to invest in your interests, in you, in your well-being." He could not possibly know how much he boosted my sense of self-worth and how it affected so much of my life. The story is not about golf, it is about relationship, about feeling good about oneself and each other, feeling valued and worthy. In time, I began to realize that this lovely man was a "God figure" to me. He reminded me of my heavenly Father. I began to read the Scripture with new eyes, eyes that unveiled a God who loves, affirms, encourages, and helps. Yes, and, when necessary, disciplines. But then discipline becomes an activity rooted in love, desiring for me the best and guiding me away from a destructive path.

Now sixty years after this story transpired, it still sticks in my mind as among the more formative in my life. It contains several levels of affect: feeling valued, good, and worthy, all of which are embodied in the word *appreciation*—the key word in the title of Level II. Keep all those words and others that touch on affect or emotion in mind as you read this chapter. Not only are they used interchangeably, but only in their particular nuances do they accumulate to express the range of affect we want to express in this chapter.

"Over the years, most teacher education classes have told prospective teachers to focus on reason, cover the curriculum, and avoid emotions in their lessons."[1] The emergence of brain research provides the evidence supporting the role of emotion—the critical role—in learning and changing.

To think of emotions as a mushy, unpredictable detriment to learning would be a serious, even dangerous oversight. And yet, that was a rather common assumption in the earlier years of education and remains in some circles. The advent of brain research brought a serious rethinking of the relationship of emotions and learning. Emotions are, in fact, the *gateway* to the kind of learning we all aspire to achieve with our students.[2]

INTRODUCING TERMS AND CONNECTIONS

Values and emotion are interwoven. What we value we feel most positive about. Additionally, we call this "Recall with Appreciation" because the valuing connects us to remembering the content. The content (Recall) creates the framework for what we value. What we judge to be negative, in error, or from poor judgment we tend to reject. Many educators tend not to use values because that implies some ideas or actions are more desirable than others. In today's world, such a stance creates heated debate. Because we anchor, to the best of our ability, our values in special revelation (the Bible) and general revelation, we believe God has made clear the values that ought to guide our thinking, feeling, and living. What we value we also love.

EMOTIONS IN PERSPECTIVE

Emotions affect memory. The more intense an emotion, positive or negative, the more likely the thought or the experience immediately enters long term memory. We never forget touching the hot stove or an extreme fright, or the first kiss or the wedding day. The body releases chemicals that place these high pain or pleasure experiences into long-term memory.

Emotion, once thought to be located in one area of the brain, is actually distributed across seven areas. Interestingly, each of these areas is activated during learning sessions, meaning that emotions and learning are very closely tied.[3]

James Zull, Professor of Biology, Biochemistry, and Cognitive Science at Case Western Reserve University forcefully states,

Emotion is probably the most important factor for learning. Our feelings determine the energy with which we begin new challenges and where we will direct that energy. The actions we take are determined by how we feel and how we believe those actions will make us feel.[4]

BRIEF OVERVIEW OF AFFECTIVE EDUCATION[5]

During the 1960s the field of *affective* education was given special attention at Michigan State University (probably other universities as well), where both of us, at different times, forged much of our educational philosophy and practice. For me (Duane) the notion that *feelings* or *emotions* (*affect*) would have a role in learning provided new insights. It was clear, even in my early twenties, that I often learned a subject better if I *liked* the teacher or the subject or both. That was true for me. It was also true that the more *respect* I *felt* from the teacher the more I wanted to learn and did *better* at learning. Still more *intriguing*, it seemed to me that others often chose subjects and even vocations that were consistent with their positive *feelings* about a certain teacher and certain classes. That was also true for me. The *pain* of a low grade, a *harsh* or *insensitive* or *boring* teacher definitely steered me in another direction. My positive *feelings* about the teacher and the topic, among other things, were major contributors toward my vocational choice. (Note all the affective words highlighted by italics in this section.)

Yet the role of emotions in learning never seemed to gain traction, at least in the mainstream of higher education except, possibly, in some pockets of the social sciences and the fine arts. Most teachers carried on as though the traditional lecture was still the most reliable method to ensure good learning. Perhaps the lack of findings from "physical sciences" contributed to a weak educational theory. No longer would this be true.

This past decade has seen major advances in cognitive, affective, and social neuroscience that have the potential to revolutionize educational theories about learning. The importance of emotion and social learning has long been recognized in education, but due to technological limitations in neuroscience research techniques, treatment of these topics in educational theory has largely not had the benefit of biological evidence to date. But there is a revolution imminent in education. The past decade has seen unprecedented advances in scientists' understanding of the brain and mind, and new information about the brain is expanding the influence of cognitive neuroscience in particular, which could have profound implications for education, eventually leading to innovations in practice and policy.[6]

WHAT'S GOING ON?

What, exactly, was going on that emotion would even affect peoples' vocational choices and learning in general? Was it just feeling good, or was more happening that might be useful in how we approach the noble goal of teaching? Positive experiences are treasured because, quite frankly, they affirm who we are as human beings. They contribute to the building of a healthy self-image, which experience and psychology tell us are foundational components to success in life.[7] For Christians, human dignity is grounded in God's unique act of creating human beings in his own image (Gen 1:26-27; 5:3; 9:6). Bearing the image or likeness of God affirms the dignity of every human being; each one is worthy of honor and respect.

Insights from the brain research as well as the social sciences increases our understanding of the teaching-learning process. For many of us, science and emotions are not used in the same sentence. Surprisingly, science now offers an explanation for why feelings must be considered not only in the classroom but every place where formal, non-formal, or informal teaching takes place: home, places of worship, small group studies, in-service training, colleges, and virtually anywhere some form of instruction occurs.

EMOTIONS AND THE BIBLE

The Bible has some surprising insights about emotions as well. While some uses of the word *feel* refer to the physical, as in touching a surface, others refer to a feeling of compassion (Heb 4:15, "For we do not have a high priest who is unable to empathize . . .") or the idea of being past feeling, i.e., callousness or insensitivity (Eph 4:19).

The Bible also uses *heart* to describe its centrality in the emotional/affective arena as well. Vine says: "The heart, in its moral significance in the Old Testament, includes the emotions, the reason and the will."[8] Vine also states that heart (*kardia*) "came to stand for man's entire mental and moral activity, both the rational and the emotional elements."[9] Thus, God wishes every part of our humanity to be brought under his authority and rule. That is why we teach; that is why we learn. Special and general revelation tell us *what* to learn. And, as we will see, our emotions determine *if* and *when* we learn. From our emotions spring behaviors.

EMOTIONS AND LEARNING

Understanding the role of emotion or feeling in education is considered by many educators to be the most important component in learning because it takes us beyond cognition, which is the stopping point for many.

Brain research has been powerful in describing the role of emotions in learning. There are several parts of the brain, called the *pleasure centers*, that respond to positive emotions. When these pleasure centers are active (positive emotions) the rational part of the brain (including reasoning, thinking, and logic) also becomes active.[10]

> *Reason seems to be always driven by emotion and need. It seems unlikely that reason could ever occur without emotion.*
>
> J. E. ZULL, *THE ART OF CHANGING THE BRAIN*

There is even evidence that an atmosphere controlled by logic may actually reduce thought and rational behavior. Jerome Kagan, a Harvard University psychologist, says,

> The rationalists who are convinced that feelings interfere with the most adaptive choices have the matter completely backwards. A reliance on logic alone, without the capacity to feel, . . . would lead most people to do many, many more foolish things.[11]

By contrast, when the fear center of the brain—the amygdala being a primary location for negative emotions—is active, the rational part of the brain tends *not* to engage except in extreme threat situations. Thus, negative emotions hijack the reasoning part of the brain and hinder learning. Damasio, a leading pioneer in emotion and learning, states that "reduction in emotion may constitute an equally important source of *irrational* behavior."[12]

Speaking about learners, Immordino-Yang and Faeth conclude that:

> If [students] feel no connection to the knowledge they learn in school, then the academic content will seem emotionally meaningless to them. Even if they manage to regurgitate factual information, it will not influence their decisions and behavior. . . . For effective cognition to manifest itself in the classroom and beyond, emotions need to be a part of the learning experience all along.[13]

Scans from fMRI studies show that when the learner's emotional state is neutral or negative, few synaptic connections show up on the monitor that measures the reasoning or thinking part of the brain. By contrast, when the learner is in a positive emotional state, the monitor shows high levels of activity (synaptic connections) in the region measuring reason or logic. In both cases, the fMRI shows the affective parts of the brain to be comparably active in both the positive and negative affective conditions. But the thinking, reasoning, and logic part of the brain activates only when the emotional state is in a more positive mode or when threat requires quick assessment and action.

Affective learning has to do with our feelings—about the class, the content, the teacher, the other learners, and even the environment. Negative feelings close the door to learning. In the classroom, negative feelings can include boredom, perceived lack of relevancy, fear of failure, embarrassment from not knowing answers, a sense the teacher does not like you or doesn't care, bullying or mockery from classmates, confusion, threat, anxiety, low grades, even conflict in the home, or the failure of a special friendship.

> *Emotions interact with reason to support or inhibit learning.*
>
> DAVID A. SOUSA, *HOW THE BRAIN LEARNS*

Positive feelings, on the other hand, open the door to learning—the kind that eventually influences behavior. Positive affect includes excitement, interest, perceived value of the information, a sense the teacher respects you as well as classmates, a sense of emotional and physical safety, and relevance of content to life. "How a person feels about a learning situation determines the amount of attention devoted to it."[14]

WHAT DOES THIS MEAN?

Learners in a negative emotional state may still memorize material, even get high marks on a test, but probably have minimal, if any, lasting learning because the rational part of the brain was minimally engaged. Thus, a student may remain in a negative state the entire class and still get an "A" for the class. But is that the kind of learning we desire?

The same student, but in a positive affective state, is more inclined to think about the material, exercise reason, and engage in dialogue—all of which moves that material from immediate to working memory. At this point, the learners begin to "own" the content and the potential for it to go into long term memory. Rita Smilkstein states in her book, *We're Born to Learn*, "Emotions produce chemicals that enter the brain and physiologically affect the synapses and, consequently, the brain's ability to think, learn, and remember. Thus, emotions, and thinking, learning, and remembering are inextricably bound together."[15]

Today, an awareness of the importance of emotions becomes a primary means by which we can be friends, healers, counselors, and guides. Traumas such as divorce in the home, addictions, depression, anxiety, mental illness, and various forms of physical and mental abuse contribute in profoundly negative ways to the way people function, perhaps more so for the younger generation but certainly all generations. At the Urbana 18 student missions conference, the top-selling books were not about missions or ministry related topics but about *anxiety*. Those who seek to nurture in the home, school, church, or community need to be aware of these often hidden emotional states that affect peoples' ability to function in life.

Here is a little exercise that will encourage the thinking part of your brain. Briefly respond to the following questions.

In your years as a student,

- what did teachers do that promoted positive affect in you? Negative affect?
- what were the outcomes of each?
- what should we be doing to create a positive atmosphere in our teaching and nurturing?

SAFETY IN OUR PRESENCE

As tensions grow in our society, we often find students feeling stressed, "out of sorts." They enter our classrooms, our pews, our dinner tables bearing emotional burdens and unable to focus on much else. Yes, they may appear to be paying attention, but there is a good chance their minds are elsewhere. What to do?

Since safety is such an important factor, we must make sure that as people come into our presence, wherever that is, they feel safe emotionally, socially, and physically. "Students must sense that the teacher *wants* to help them rather than catch them being wrong."[16]

We promote safety when we greet them by name, smile, inquire as to their well-being, show respect, spend extra time before and after class and, as some of my professor friends do, invite students over to our houses for an evening or meet them one-on-one for lunch, breakfast, or just to talk. My former students, after twenty and even thirty years, reflect fondly on those social times, private times, times we shared life together. If the brain research is correct, more happened than just good socializing: the sense of well-being opened the door for deeper learning, the kind God uses to transform us into his image. And that is what my golfing friend did for me, by God's grace.

Golfing is not the way most of us can reach out to students, but let's ask this question: "What can I do to make the students feel more safe with me?"[17] For the sake of our students, parishioners, children, neighbors, let's ponder the answer.

Dave does several things to build safety with his students. Early on in his courses, he has each student set up an hour lunch time with him. This signals immediately that each one is important. He begins lunch by asking them, "Tell me about yourself." Usually, that consumes the entire time. The giving of time in the academic world is a powerful message. Then Dave has each class to his house for an

> *Emotion is our biological thermostat and is thus central to cognition and . . . practice.*
>
> ROBERT SYLVESTER

evening around food and getting to know one another. Last, he arrives early to class to greet every person and stays after to be available for any who want to talk further. Is it any wonder students gravitate toward him anytime he walks the campus?

CREDIBILITY OF THE TEACHER

There are two types of credibility: *competence* credibility, also called professional competence, which means students and others trust us to do our job well. The second is *safety* credibility, also called relational credibility. Can we be trusted with their story—be it pain, success, or something simpler, like the need to talk? Do our students feel safe to approach us? It is not a question of whether *we* feel safe for others to approach us, but do *they* feel safe? Some university professors in Central and Eastern Europe have no office hours (or no office). Some schools have only commuters who live at a distance. Still others take courses online. The challenge for each is how to build "safety credibility" with students in these circumstances.

We are not saying that a given teacher can and must earn the trust of everyone and that everyone must feel safe with a teacher. That would not allow for the variety of personalities. But if a given teacher is never, or rarely, approached by someone with a personal concern, that may indicate the safety or trust level is not strong. All of us need to think about this, for we are all people who wish to minister not only to the mind but to the whole person.

Students must feel physically safe and emotionally secure before they can focus on the curriculum.

DAVID A. SOUSA, *HOW THE BRAIN LEARNS*

Teachers are role models and therefore need to model both professionalism and the personal, the relational. Seminaries have a reputation for outstanding, competent faculty. They are impressive in their scholarship and lecturing. However, since the mission of most seminaries is the training of pastors and Christian leaders, the success of their graduates will depend at least as much on the graduates' ability to connect relationally with their congregations as their ability to do scholarly preaching. How well the seminary graduate cares for people may be perceived as being as important as the polished sermon. Training shepherds and training scholars should be co-equal goals.

A good example was Dave (above) who, in building trust and becoming safe with students, was also being pastoral. Periodically I would ask former students what they remembered about their time on campus. Two answers dominated: the professors and the informal times. Regarding professors, the primary characteristic was friendliness, willingness to talk and "hang out." To that end, one campus paid for the professors' lunch if they would meet with a student or students. Friendliness (safety) emerged as a school value. (And yes, some former students mentioned outstanding lectures and competent faculty, positive and necessary attributes to be sure.)

Here is my own effort at being pastoral. Regarding the informal times, I had students over for evenings at our house as well. Years later those informal times are the first memories they recall. But I also made sure that if a student was an athlete or musician or in some extracurricular activity, I would attend at least one event that semester. Then I would mention it to the student as I saw them on campus or as they entered the next class. It often began a conversation.

Some students seemed less easy to connect with. I then tried to find something in their paper assignments and asked them if they could expand on it for my own benefit. "Teaching" the teacher rarely failed to inspire the quieter ones to engage with me.

Walking the halls of our Christian colleges can be a revealing exercise. Some professors have sign-up sheets on their doors. On one campus I noticed that the sign-up time slots were for fifteen minutes. On another campus the time slots were for half-hour segments. This signaled a difference from my perspective. In fifteen minutes, the professor has time to answer a few questions. With a brief time slot, the student can easily feel the "business" needs to be brief and official. In thirty minutes, the student may feel less pressure to be quick and precise. Additionally, the professor can move beyond answers to discussion and trust-building. Am I making too much of this? I wonder.

SELF-CONCEPT (SELF-IMAGE) AND LEARNING

Self-concept is the sum of all our experiences that have impacted how we view ourselves. Self-concept (sometimes called self-worth, self-esteem, or ego strength) can be high or low or anywhere in between. We all have a self-concept and it affects us every day in all our relationships and in our learning. Self-concept may be more positive if we have had more successful experiences and encouragement from people in our lives. Or the opposite could be true. Creating positive, successful experiences may cancel out some of the undesirable experiences and build a better image of self. The educator can assist by making sure the learning environment contains positive experiences.[18]

For another example, I (Duane) use lots of questions and activities in my classes. I make it a habit never to criticize a student. If someone makes a sincere comment but it really represents poor judgment, misinformation, or dislocated logic, I acknowledge the comment, thank the person for sharing their thought and try to remember several really important things:

- The student made an honest effort; that should not be discouraged.

- If I make them feel stupid, there is a good chance that will be the last comment they make for a long while; furthermore, they likely will not hear the correct or better information since a negative emotion (embarrassment? failure?) will block learning; people with high self-esteem may not be so susceptible to failure.

- I try to come back to their comment later with a slightly different but more correct spin saying, "I think this is what so-and-so was getting at earlier," to which the learner nearly always gives a happy nod.

- I will be especially sensitive to international students who are working in their second, third, or fourth language and may not be as articulate as a native English speaker; they embarrass more easily if told they are wrong or even just get the feeling they may have been wrong.

Those who have been criticized or scolded in past class settings bring fear if not dread to the next class. I work hard to avoid this; I want them to feel welcome, valued, accepted—that they are an important contributor to everyone else present. Under these conditions the brain eagerly invites new thoughts, expansive ideas, and growth.

> *Emotional states have a pervasive influence on learning.*
>
> ERIC JENSEN, *TEACHING WITH THE BRAIN IN MIND*

I've heard teachers say, "I limit discussion because students only share their ignorance." Since ignorance is what you don't know, you cannot share what you don't know. What they may share is misinformation, incomplete knowledge, or errant thinking. Is it not better to know what is in their minds so that you can, at a minimum, share your own perspective? If we disparage student answers or comments, that may be the end of hearing from them. Furthermore, the bitter feeling (yes, that negative emotion) may only serve to cement that errant thought in their mind.

People who have had negative learning experiences in the past often enter our classrooms fearful, guarded, and reticent—all negative emotions. Or if they have come into our classrooms just having broken up with a close friend, experienced their parents in a fight, been bullied by peers, or just discovered they have a serious illness, these emotions will dominate their mind and our words may enter their computer notes but not their minds. And as noted above, those emotions will probably inhibit their capacity to think and reason—to process class material—making them less motivated to learn.[19] For the most part, that material will be lost forever. It will not even enter working memory. So what can be done?[20]

Those are not improbable situations; we might think they are, but that is only because we do not know our students that well. We just see them as students taking notes, coming and going with only class assignments and tests on their minds. Here is what we can—must—do. If our students walk into our classrooms and feel safe, valued, accepted, wanted, honored, privileged, and welcomed by all, the negative feelings dissipate for the moment and allow the learner to engage. Even better, if they are free to share their need and have someone pray for them, they can set that concern aside, having given it to their loving Father while feeling the loving support of their learning community—including you, especially you!

From Negative to Positive Experiences

No one enjoys disappointment or failure. These experiences are, however, inevitable. At such times, if the teacher has built a positive relationship and a positive learning environment, correction will be received as an act of care rather than rejection or failure.

There will be times when the student will simply not be able to perform for whatever reason. Every effort has been extended to help the learner succeed but nothing has worked. Again, if the relationship is strong, the learner will see the teacher's efforts and realize that the teacher's identification of failure has, in fact, been a favor. Now the learner is free to think of an alternative. The lessons the learner may walk away with are several:

1. The teacher respects me and works hard for my success, but this is just "not my thing."

2. When I teach, I want to honor my students in the same way.

3. I may have failed but I am not a failure.

The brain literature calls this "role modeling."[21] Creating a supportive, positive emotional environment may be the most important lesson students carry away whether in success or (temporary) failure.

The Power of Story

Stories are among the more powerful techniques for learning. Similar techniques include one's own experience, short readings from a book, case studies, biography, metaphors, and analogies.[22] But what makes story a powerful form of learning? Zull states,

Stories engage all parts of the brain. . . . They allow us to package events and knowledge in complex neuronal nets, any part of which can trigger all the others. And stories are about movement. They focus on good and bad actions, so they generate fear and pleasure, and all the derivative emotions.[23]

Since stories are packaged as "whole experiences," they are easier to remember as are details of the story including emotions, lessons learned, and the desire to repeat the story, resulting in deeper learning.

Zull illustrates this point about deeper learning with a story about algebra concluding with "a moral. Algebra is about fairness. . . . Learning is about life. Stories bring things to life and life into things."[24]

Robert Coles, a Harvard professor of psychology, teaches his classes through story. Harvard Law School makes prolific use of case studies. As this information became known to me years ago, I determined to try it in one of my classes. I used three books, two of which were biography (each representing a different view of cultural engagement) and one of which was more theory-based. The undergraduate students guided the discussion. Prior to each class, the team of

> *Stories engage all parts of the brain.*
>
> J.A. ZULL, *THE ART OF CHANGING THE BRAIN*

students (usually two) met with me to go over their class plan. During class time I participated (rather sparingly) along with the others. At the end, many said it was the best class they had experienced to that point in their college program. Discussion prompts emotions and values to surface in the conscious mind where reflection, evaluation and, potentially, change can occur. Story seems to stimulate thought more effectively than virtually any other form, save for personal experience.

Traveling stateside and abroad, I often use a metaphorical story about a monkey and a fish.

> A typhoon had temporarily stranded a monkey on an island. In a secure, protected place, while waiting for the raging waters to recede, he spotted a fish swimming against the current. It seemed obvious to the monkey that the fish was struggling and in need of assistance. Being of kind heart, the monkey resolved to help the fish.
>
> A tree precariously dangled over the very spot where the fish seemed to be struggling. At considerable risk to himself, the monkey moved far out on a limb, reached down and snatched the fish from the threatening waters. Immediately scurrying back to the safety of his shelter, he carefully laid the fish on dry ground. For a few moments the fish showed excitement, but soon

settled into a peaceful rest. Joy and satisfaction swelled inside the monkey. He had successfully helped another creature.[25]

I used this story in Bangladesh with a group of community development workers. The discussion was animated during debriefing, where open questions were posed. But more important, two years later when my wife was back in the same area doing further work, a Bangladeshi leader sidled up to her and whispered, "I'm not like the monkey." Two years later that story still guided his interactions with others.

SUMMARY

Emotions signal what we value or, in the case of negative emotions, what we fear or dislike. Most of our choices are grounded in some emotion: positive emotions draw us in and open the mind to learn; situations that surface negative emotions we will tend to avoid and close the door to processing information. The teacher's ability to create a safe environment in the classroom will affect how people feel, think, and respond. We can be a haven of safety, affirmation, encouragement, and good teaching practices that give learners every opportunity to succeed in their endeavors.

Jensen makes this clear:

> Neuroscientists are breaking new ground in helping us understand why emotion is an important learning variable, and how the affective side of learning is the critical interplay between how we feel, act, and think. Mind and emotions are not separate; emotions, thinking, and learning are all linked. What we feel *is* what's real—even if only to us and no one else. Emotions organize and create our reality.[26]

Eyler uses a metaphor to help us understand emotion and learning:

> Most of the time emotion and cognition cooperate quite nicely. Each needs the other, as dance partners do, in order to follow the choreography that leads to deep learning. Instructors can use this partnership to our advantage as we create assignments and activities that harness emotion for pedagogical gain.[27]

LEVEL 3

Recall with Speculation

I ponder how to use the information

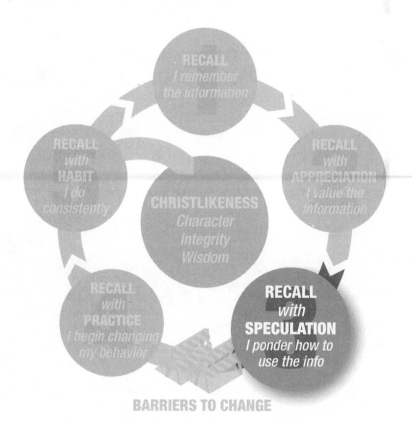

CHAPTER SIX

From Content to Experience

Blessed rather are those who hear the word of God and obey it.

JESUS, LUKE 11:28

The belief that people change just by listening to a sermon could be one of the most detrimental naiveties in our church today.

KYLE STROBEL *METAMORPHA: JESUS AS A WAY OF LIFE*

Transfer is the basis of all creativity, problem solving, and the making of satisfying decisions.

MADELINE HUNTER, *MASTERY TEACHING*

S PECULATION, AS WE ARE USING IT, refers to the intentional reflection on some aspect of content with the purpose of discovering what it means for one's own life. Some authors prefer *transfer* or *transferability*. We will treat them as synonyms.[1] Speculation includes (a) interpreting new situations more accurately with new knowledge, (b) being able to apply new knowledge to solve problems, and (c) being able to creatively use new knowledge to engage people and events more productively.

In our adult Sunday school class, we all made a commitment to attend the middle worship service and then attend the class afterwards. The purpose of our class was to discuss the sermon. More specifically we intended two objectives: (1) name the sermon content from which God spoke to us or made something memorable and (2) identify how that content might impact our life—or, in what way (or ways) that truth might change us to be better kingdom representatives of our Lord. The leaders acted as facilitators, not deliverers of content. The sermon was our content. Our small numbers, averaging around fifteen or sixteen, made this class structure very doable.[2] The consistent attendance suggested people enjoyed this format. Comments from week to week indicated people were applying and growing.

Using content from another source (i.e., the sermon) and then discussing and applying it in community (i.e., our Sunday school class) helped us take application seriously. Knowing we would be discussing the sermon later motivated us to pay closer attention, take notes, and look for thoughts that would impact our lives. Since the hypocrite factor resides within each of us, we did not relax our efforts to eradicate its beastly presence.

But what of our students in the physical and social sciences, our children at the dinner table, the congregation? How might we help them deal with their own gravitation to wander from the good? The Learning Cycle considers this important step with understanding and help for the teacher.

Prone to wander, Lord, I feel it. Prone to leave the God I love.

ROBERT ROBINSON, "COME THOU FOUNT OF EVERY BLESSING"

Educators must be intentional about helping learners speculate on how they might use the information. Such intentionality is necessary for promoting outcomes. The same holds for those in mentoring, discipling, Bible study lessons, family devotions, or whatever form your teaching takes. Failure to honor speculation as a legitimate teaching activity and worthy of space in your curriculum may result in serious lapses in building habits of faith.

SPECULATION STARTS WITH A BRAIN CONNECTION

In brain science terms, speculation (transfer) is defined as that which occurs when new information connects with past information and prompts the learner to imagine what might be. Or in briefer terms, transfer is attempting to answer the "So what?" question after encountering and reflecting on a body of content.[3]

Speculation presumes that one can transfer learning to life. The ability to speculate about the potential of new knowledge looms large in the brain literature for one simple reason: if we cannot visualize how information can be transferred to life situations, we will never improve, never grow, never advance. It makes goal setting futile and learning fruitless. The inability to transfer content to new situations serves to merely reinforce one's own mistaken beliefs and ineffectual behaviors, that is, to try to solve new problems with our old ways of thinking and believing.

Speculation involves three transactions on the part of the learner: (1) thinking about relevant information (working memory), (2) connecting it with past content (in long-term memory), and (3) beginning to speculate (future) about appropriate action.

Let's see how this works out with a recent concern of mine: the way politicians, and many people in general (including myself) have been using degrading or dehumanizing language about anyone who disagrees with their respective beliefs. Plenty of guilt can be found on either side. Christians also engage in this practice, demonizing the other side without conscience. Since I am responsible for my thinking, I decided to do something about my problem.

I ask, *Is there an ethic or moral code that I should be referencing?* So I search for scriptural guidance. *How do I connect my present understanding of this problem with content that will help me move forward?* So I read, "Those who guard their mouths and their tongues keeps themselves from calamity" (Prov 21:23). The psalmist says good days accompany those who "keep [their] tongue from evil" (Ps 34:13), a thought reinforced in 1 Peter 3:10. Paul exhorts, "rid yourselves of . . . malice, slander, and filthy language from your lips" (Col 3:8). Rather, Paul continues, "Let your conversation be always full of grace" (Col 4:6). I also review my understanding of the image of God (Jas 3:9) and realize some of my language violates the belief that language is one way we nudge people toward eternal glory . . . or the opposite.[4] So now I have connected my present situation with past learning—recall from long term memory.

But now comes speculation. *What is the appropriate action? How do I make this happen?* In this case, it is obvious: keep my mouth shut. But that will require other actions if I am to be successful. I will need to monitor my thoughts, evaluate their value and fitness to the situation. If they are slanderous, degrading, or filthy, I must resist thinking or speaking them. If, however, I wish to speak into a situation, then it must be done with grace, honesty, and without slander. This will require more thought and careful crafting of language in a day that knows little of constraint. In pursuing this new challenge, my discipline to manage this process has been severely tested. I find myself failing with shocking regularity. I am a person of opinion, quick words, and—too frequently—limited control of my tongue. I have not succeeded . . . yet! But I continue to work on it. I am making progress. And, I will persevere. (Sometimes stubbornness can work to one's advantage.)

Zull adds several more parallel terms corresponding to speculation (or transfer): imaging, problem solving, prediction, vision, and future thinking.[5] Thus, as noted earlier, unless learners can actually "see" a way to use content they will be unable to solve problems, evaluate situations, critique ideas or use what they have learned to transact life beyond the classroom. They may get "A's" on all the tests but flunk life—that is, unless they can speculate on the possible uses of an important body of content.

We use speculation to signal the point at which content becomes part of our thinking and produces a possibility of actions culminating in a decision to act. It would be accurate to say of someone who has acquired lots of facts that the person "is very knowledgeable" or "scholarly" or even "well informed." These terms accurately described the Pharisees and teachers of the law. But given our understanding of *learning*, one could not say that they had learned the Scripture since they had not lived in accordance with it.

LEARNING TASKS TO ENSURE SPECULATION

Zull expounds on the need for mingling speculation and action—new knowledge leading to speculation leading to experience (action).[6] To accomplish this, in my Cross-Cultural Ministry class, I would send my students to connect with people in the nearby immigrant community. At other times we would be on the streets of the inner city or in an immigrant church; or helping in a community center or prison. Sometimes, however, these may not be available or the right kind of experience we wish for our students. When a "real" situation was not available, we found case studies and video clips to be very productive.

Zull also makes a strong point about the role of talking, which he believes to be "possibly the most fundamental of all" the components in a learning task. "But the one essential condition is that the talking should be useful talk. Talk that explains, that questions, that invents new ideas, that motivates." It must be focused and accompanied by "active listening."[7] But, continues Zull,

"Another way to nurture problem solving and critical thinking is writing. . . . It is permanent. It can be reconsidered later, when we might forget the talk. And it is slower. It facilitates more reflection and more careful thought."[8] Remember our assignment to write a "memo to myself" (chapter three)? It also promotes reflective thought and transfer.

In our culture and ministry classes, we found a book that had seventy cultural situations in which the students had to solve or explain a cultural dilemma. Usually they would get it wrong or mostly wrong because they tried to solve the problem from their own cultural framework (old knowledge). Eventually they would have new knowledge available to them and then we would see if they could solve a different but similar problem using the new knowledge. Given enough practice, we found that students grew quite adept at choosing good responses. Furthermore, the different cultural dilemmas created an enthusiastic problem-solving atmosphere where students enjoyed seeing if they could suggest appropriate responses. When they could, we had reasonable assurance that they had learned because they could speculate from what they had learned to a new situation and correctly discern (speculate) the proper response.

But it is not always so easy. We found speculation more difficult with undergraduates because their experience base was more limited. Case studies, videos, and field trips were necessary and most helpful. Personal illustrations and biography were also popular ways of bringing a vicarious experience into their lives. Graduate students usually had more experience and could speculate how they would have done something differently given the new knowledge derived from the textbook, the lecture, class discussion, or some other source. They speculated how it could have been and, if they enter similar situations in the future, how they will handle it differently—a very legitimate reflection-speculation combination.

FROM CONTENT MASTERY TO SPECULATION

In my Human Development and Learning class, I had the learners do a comparison of major learning theorists. For each they had to side by side put the theorist's view of knowledge, of learning, of educational process, of the role of the teacher (professor), and, finally, of the role of the learner. All of this was done in groups of three or four and would be summarized in one to two pages and in columns for ease of comparison. In class each group shared their responses.

Members were encouraged to change their answers if they heard something better. The last piece of the activity was to briefly evaluate each theorist from a Christian worldview based on the framework of the Scripture. They were to work with the assumption that each theorist would have something to contribute to our view of learning and something that would not be acceptable to the Christian mind and practice. Last, they were to write a brief summary of how they might improve their own teaching ministry (speculation based on new knowledge).

This activity accomplished several things: the learners had to read, write, summarize, and evaluate core teachings of theorists. Each step required thought (i.e., recall of past/recent learning brought into working memory). The evaluative part forced them to reflect on their own Christian framework for discernment. Sharing with others (more working memory, further strengthening the neural network) forced them to articulate for the benefit of others (creating sense and meaning for others). The feedback each gave to the others (again, working memory) further strengthened the neural pathway (or corrected it).

The last piece of the activity was each group sharing while I put their respective answers on the white board. As each piece of the information was shared, it was open to critique by the class and myself. At the end we had a huge white board full of major theorists and their respective views on core learning precepts.

The last part of the activity above was reflecting on ones' own teaching pattern. Given this new knowledge,

- what part of my teaching may be weak?
- how should I change to be more effective? (What should I do differently?)
- what is the basis for this change? (What new knowledge prompts this change?)
- what are my expectations in making this change? (What do I want to see?)

Later, Muriel used this same summarizing technique with her graduate level class, Adult Education Theorists. At the end of the class, all the summaries were posted on newsprint around the room. The students walked around the room looking at each summary (rehearsal) and then wrote a "memo to myself" speculating on what they planned to incorporate into their own teaching.

When learners begin to see multiple applications for a concept they now understand and perceive as relevant, learning motivation increases and the brain is energized for more stimulation. Knowledge is power and the best exercise of that power is the ability to solve problems—especially if the problems had been perplexing and had defied resolution.

In an attempt to get a Sunday school class of high school juniors to think about the meaning of "church," I asked them to write every word that came to mind when they heard the word *church*. Some chuckled or giggled as they wrote. The lists were quite long. Their next assignment was to put a single line through (but not obliterate) every item on the list that could not be supported by Scripture, either a verse or a biblical concept. Then I passed out a series of questions, each of which elicited discussion:

- What did you learn from this exercise?
- What accounts for the items you put a line through? Where did they come from and/or why are they part of our church practice?
- What would church look like if we eliminated all the items you scratched out?
- How would you change "church" if given the chance to do so? Who would most value the change(s)? Are there people who would not value the change(s)? How should that influence your decision(s)?

While they found the exercise intriguing, even a bit amusing, they were hesitant and guarded about what they would do differently. Being high school juniors, this would have been new thinking and they were unprepared to offer critique. Yet their lists revealed that over two-thirds of the words they wrote when presented with the word *church* were actually not found in the Bible, based on their present thinking. They were warned not to think of something as unbiblical simply because it could not be found in the Bible. Rather, every worshipping group surrounds itself with forms that provide meaning as that group enters corporate worship. We call those forms *tradition*, and those pieces of our worship should be examined but not arbitrarily tossed out.

GALLUP ON LEARNING AND PERCEPTION OF RELEVANCE

A Gallup poll of over 900,000 middle school and high school students revealed that as students progressed through the grades, they became less and less engaged with the content. [9] The reason? Their teachers failed to impress on them the future importance of the content. Sousa states: "If students do not perceive how the information or skill can be used for the future, they will tend to pay little attention and exert even less effort."[10] In other words, little impact on behavior occurs without intentional effort by the teachers to (1) connect the importance of the content to life, (2) provide space for students to process more deeply the content (rehearsal), and (3) encourage each to think specifically about how the content might affect their own behavior (speculation).

The easiest thing in the world is to take notes in class and set them aside until the test. It is common to the point of being axiomatic. For sure, it is an unintended consequence—an unintended habit—we have instilled by default. And it cripples many who naively believe they are growing in the Christian life only to realize the growth is largely cognitive with little effect on their character development.

Certainly teachers and, in our opinion, most students really want their lives and their faith to grow stronger, more robust, more clearly aligned with God's own will. Furthermore, they expect this outcome as a result of being in our classes. Is it possible we have unwittingly abdicated a key role in teaching— bringing the learners to discern how God's truth is intended to impact life?

While Muriel was teaching nursing, she helped to create a new medical surgical curriculum for the university that made speculation imperative. Before coming to class, the nursing students were expected to read and watch videos that covered all the class content. Class time was not used to go over content that they had already covered. In class, then, they were presented with a case study of a patient with the same diagnosis as their study material. They were expected to speculate and apply what they had already learned to the case-study patient. In the following two days they were assigned a real patient in the hospital with that diagnosis and had to present a nursing care plan to the instructor for the care of that patient the following day.

We are convinced that learners need to be taught to speculate on how content should be consistently applied to real world problems. This is true for any discipline be it biology, accounting, literature, history, or any other, though one might argue especially for biblical truth. For teachers, it's a serious responsibility. It is not just nice or helpful. It is critical in today's world where there are so many problems to be solved and lives to be transformed. Teachers cannot abandon their learners to travel from theory to practice alone. There are a multitude of teaching techniques they can use to motivate learners to think about how an idea could address a real problem. These include problem-based learning, case studies, simulations, instructional games, and just good old open questions about how an idea applies to practice. These techniques move ideas into working memory, where they establish stronger neural networks and ultimately enhance the probability that learners will act on what they are learning.

An Unholy Habit—Unintended Consequences

Could it be that the "great escape" may refer not only to students failing to ponder the meaning of classroom material; could it also describe those of us who have "escaped" the responsibility of nurturing contemplation, meaning-making, and the will to change as a necessary step in teaching? By ignoring this crucial learning activity, by being too preoccupied with packing in more content, we "tell" people that it is not important, it is not necessary, and it can be skipped. In other words, we have unknowingly created an unholy habit by which our learners skip the connection between truth and life. While emphasizing the knowing (cognition) of truth, we inadvertently teach them that the practice of truth is not important or as important.

This unintended consequence takes us to the very center of the problem, that which began this journey: unholy habits may account for so much of the hypocrisy we see in the church, Bible schools, seminaries, and the faith community at large. Teachers shudder at the thought, and we all wish it were not so. But read on.

Truth is barren when not connected to life experience. It remains an idea void of personal meaning or application. As such, the idea dies quickly because the brain discards meaningless or disconnected thoughts.[11] But reflecting on an idea, followed by speculating on the "So what?" introduces the learner to the potential of truth and its purpose: to become more Christlike. "What does God want me to do with what I am learning?" is the chief concern of speculation. Furthermore, the very act of thinking ahead grows the neural network, making it more robust and accessible for future connections.[12]

Truth (content) bears fruit when learners reflect on that which the Holy Spirit has impressed upon their minds (Level I) and hearts by way of conviction or encouragement (Level II) and a sense that this truth has consequences for living the Christian faith (Level III). Thus, the learner ponders: "Given this truth, How should I change?"

Change can take four forms:

- We *add* something that is missing in our life.

- We *modify* an existing behavior but now make it more aligned with Scripture.

- We *eliminate* a behavior that dishonors God.

- We *strengthen* an already healthy behavior to become even stronger.

The reasoning part of the brain integrates the information, makes sense of it, and waits for the next step: What to do? When learners speculate, the brain now processes at yet another level: the level of the future, "what might be." A new neural pathway begins forming and strengthens as the learner ponders. For the Christian, all responsible change emanates from the prompting of the Holy Spirit but a friend, teacher, parent, pastor, mentor, or just quiet meditation may be the instrument by which the Holy Spirit works. It often comes in the form of conviction but may also be a simple awareness. Whatever the cause, the teacher needs to create space for reflective thought about the "So what?" question.

> *If students do not perceive how the information or skill can be used for the future, they will tend to pay little attention and exert even less effort.*
>
> DAVID A. SOUSA, *HOW THE BRAIN LEARNS*

LOVE, COURTSHIP, AND MISERY: ILLUSTRATING SPECULATION

I taught a Sunday school class of high school juniors in a large church. The guidebook listed two lessons on marriage coming up. The lesson material seemed unlikely to capture their interest, so I tried my own approach. When the twenty or so juniors came in, they were told to take an index card from the table in front of me. Each card had a large letter on it: an "H" or "U" or "D." After a brief introduction I told the class the H represented a happy marriage, the U an unhappy marriage and the D a broken marriage (divorce or separation). Of course, they were all looking at the letter in their hands.

Next, I had the H's stand in one corner of the room, U's in another, and D's in yet a third corner. At that time the statistical data showed that 50 percent of the new marriages ended in divorce (D). So half the group stood together in their respective corner. The data for Christian divorce was marginally better but not at the level of statistical significance.

The unhappy marriages, while more difficult to determine, was estimated at 25 percent, though most research estimated higher. That left 25 percent in the happy marriage corner.

Everyone looked at each other as I explained the percentages. At this point, they were asked to share their observations. Comments like, "It seems almost impossible to have a happy marriage," or, "Marriage seems really hard," or, "I can't believe it's so difficult."

Next I put the U's (approximately five) together with the D's (approximately ten) so now the fifteen U's and D's were looking at the five H's. They were quite incredulous as they tried to wrap their heads around this stunning confrontation with reality.

After a moment to absorb the situation, I put them in smaller groups. With about ten in the divorced group, they worked in small groups. The other groups were similarly divided. Their assignment was to write on their index cards their answers to the question, "What contributed to the status of the marriage represented on your card?" So the D's wrote about what they thought contributed to the divorce. The U's wrote about what contributed to their condition, and so on. For the first four to five minutes, I had them write their own thoughts with no discussion. Then they had another few minutes to discuss within their own group.

After about ten to fifteen minutes, I had them share what they wrote. I recorded their comments on large sheets of newsprint each with a D or U or H at the top. They did not know this yet, but these sheets would be used the following week. They were eager to share what they had written, and the newsprint sheets filled up. I pondered where they were getting this information. It occurred to me they were, to some extent, describing their own homes and maybe others they had visited. That was all we could accomplish for one lesson, but the room buzzed as they walked out.

The following week we rehearsed what we experienced the previous week, looking at the newsprint and even adding a couple more items to the bulging lists. Then came another assignment: this time in random small groups, answer this question, "What does the Bible teach us about how to have a happy marriage?" The students were asked to be ready to explain or elaborate on their answers. Each group was given four or five Scripture references from which to build their answers. They worked for about twelve to fifteen minutes and then shared. Again, I put their responses up on newsprint. Such interest I have rarely seen.

At the end of the second session, I asked everyone to write (on smaller cards) how they may think differently or what they may do differently given the information. At my request, they made two copies of their response, one of which they would leave with me if they wished. All gave me their second card. All wrote meaningful responses, but one girl made what surely was a life-changing decision. She wrote, "As a result of this class I have decided not to elope with my boyfriend."[13]

I knew what this one girl wrote because I noticed she erased something, and her card was the only one with erasure. One never knows how God is speaking to people. That is why learning is a highly personalized experience.[14]

I lectured very little in those two sessions, but I gave the students space to talk and think about how truth is or should be influencing their decisions and behaviors with regard to marriage. In those spaces, God spoke. Failure to provide that space may mute God's voice at a critical moment when a person is listening. At the end of the year, several volunteered their comments after my last time with them: "I like the way you teach;" "I learned a lot;" "I'm sorry you

Speculation allows time to imagine my future.

DUANE ELMER

won't be with us next year;" and one that I especially prize: "I learned more in the past nine months than all the other years I have been in Sunday School combined . . . and I started in the cradle room." That comment startled me for this reason: I had done less talking in this class than any previous one. Yet they learned more. How does that work? I am hopeful the reading of this book will provide you with an answer, maybe answers. Truth be told, I was the one on a steep learning curve. Their willingness to engage, trust, and wrestle with me on issues taught me the importance of listening, questioning, clarifying, probing, dialogue, consolidating lessons learned, and pushing us to imagine.

BEAUTIFUL, COURAGEOUS LYNN

In the Sunday school story immediately above, a female junior sat silent every week. Lynn appeared interested but never spoke. One Sunday the discussion was especially animated with many jumping in to offer their thoughts. Suddenly the room became silent and as I looked around to see what might explain this strange twist, there was Lynn with her hand up. Delighted to see this, I said, "Hey Lynn, what have you got to say?" Again, silence prevailed in the room. Then, after a brief moment, Lynn began to speak. As she did, I began to understand. Lynn stuttered. With struggle she kept going, finally getting her thought out. Everyone seemed as shocked as I was. I thanked her for her contribution as I tended to do regularly.

After class one member came to me and said, "Today you made history." "What do you mean?" I replied.

He recounted a piece of history: "I have been with Lynn in every Sunday school class since we were babies, in every grade school and high school class . . . all of them we ended up together. This is the first time I have ever heard her speak in public."

Simply raising questions prompts thought and sometimes dissonance. Questions capture the attention of the brain like virtually no other teaching technique. Hoffeld says:

> Behavioral scientists have also found that just asking people about their future decisions significantly influences those decisions, a phenomenon known as the "mere measurement effect." Back in 1993, social scientists Vicki Morwitz, Eric Johnson, and David Schmittlein conducted a study with more than 40,000 participants that revealed that simply asking someone if people were going to purchase a new car within six months increased their purchase rates by 35%.
>
> So why do questions have such influence on the decision-making process?
>
> First and foremost, they prompt the brain to contemplate a behavior, which increases the probability that it will be acted upon. In fact, decades of research has [sic] found that the more the brain contemplates a behavior, the more likely it is that we will engage in it.
>
> When scientists used functional magnetic resonance imaging (MRI), they found that questions that asked participants to disclose their opinions increased neural activity in the areas of the brain associated with reward and pleasure.[15]

What caused Lynn to force unwilling words from her mouth, risking embarrassment and humiliation from her peers, as stuttering often did in those days? Lynn was so consumed with the excitement of thinking and the possibility that she could meaningfully contribute to the conversation, she cast fear to the wind and spoke—her bravery winning the respect of her peers.

We rob students of the joy of imagining and envisioning if we do not give opportunity for expressing their own story, their own thoughts, as God gives them insight and vision. And we rob ourselves of joy by not hearing the story God is authoring for each one. One of the most important roles of the teacher is drawing cohesive conclusions by raising questions; allowing for thought and cognitive dissonance; and hearing from various people. None of this negates the lecture; in fact, given a chance, well-designed questions and guided discussion will make the lecture more memorable.

RESISTANCE TO TRANSFER—IT CAN BE HARD TO CHANGE

Some years ago a Ukrainian woman, head of a linguistics department in a local university, and her husband wanted me to meet their Orthodox priest. As we drove through Kyiv, the priest and I sat in the back seat of the car conversing. He met the image that I had of Orthodox priests: older, full beard, bushy head of hair, and layers of cleric garb. Somewhere in the conversation he mentioned the youth in his country. So I asked how the church is adjusting to meet the needs of this emerging generation. Without hesitation he responded, "The Orthodox church has not changed in over five hundred years."

> *If there is no struggle, there is no progress.*
>
> FREDERICK DOUGLASS

One could deduce two possible answers to that comment: (1) "Yes, the church does not change its message," or (2) "One does not need to change methods with the changing times." While I did not press his comment, I did sense from his tone that he felt quite absolute in both respects: we do not change our content or methods. This may not represent Orthodox tradition as a whole, since one can find this view across the spectrum of Christianity.

The Pharisees and teachers of the law held a similar attitude. No need to change. We are fine just the way we are. For whatever reasons, they never got the most important part of the learning process, transferring their scriptural knowledge into consistent behaviors; that part seemed to have escaped them. Jesus, in his opening discourse, the Sermon on the Mount, warns "do not be like the hypocrites" (Mt 6:5). Change, growing into the image of Christ is what life is all about.

Summary

The concept of *speculation* helps us move beyond the Pharisees. It was the missing ingredient that would have transformed them into good shepherds who modeled a life of word and deed. The decision to speculate begins with content (Level I). What of God's truth is most important? This truth, usually accompanied by emotional energy (Level II), continues with a desire to change (Level III). All of these, of course, fall under the guidance and power of the Holy Spirit. Responsible change, governed by the Holy Spirit, occurs when there is a felt need (dissonance), discernment (reflection), and a mental picture (imagination) of what should be. These can be a part of our classroom or anywhere we offer instructional help to someone.

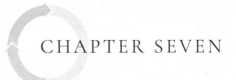

CHAPTER SEVEN

The Power of Cognitive Dissonance

*For merely listening to the law doesn't make us right with God. It
is obeying the law that makes us right in his sight.*

ROMANS 2:13 (NLT)

Emotion is our biological thermostat and is thus central to cognition and . . . practice.

ROBERT SYLVESTER

The measure of intelligence is the ability to change.

ALBERT EINSTEIN

S EVERAL WEEKS AGO I got a call from Valerie, a first year student at a
university in the Eastern United States. She was a missionary kid
("MK") from Latin America. She had a class project and asked if she
could interview me. I knew her parents and agreed happily. Since I had never
met her, I wanted a bit of background. In the process of talking, I asked,
"What do you want to be doing ten to twenty years from now?"

She replied rather quickly: "I want to help teachers teach better."

"Why are you interested in this kind of career?" I asked.

Without hesitation she answered, "Because I had some poor teachers in
my school, and I want to help them do better."

To this I asked, "Do you mind telling me what classes these poor
teachers taught?"

"They were all Bible classes," she blurted not with disgust but with deep concern—a concern that now gives direction to her career.

I was saddened. This should never happen, especially with Bible classes. From what we know from chapter five on the role of emotions and learning, we might surmise that it would have been difficult for students to enjoy and profit from such classes. The dissonance Valerie expressed was *how can poor teaching be tolerated, especially when the content is the Bible—or any other subject, for that matter?* I salute Valerie because instead of avoiding the problem, she has plunged into solving it.

Truth is paramount for the Christian. God's truth, applied by the Holy Spirit, will create dissonance in life's journey. It usually happens when God disrupts our status quo and alerts us to replacing "what is" with "what ought to be." Dissonance, difficult as it may be, is one way God grows us. With it comes disturbing ambiguity. We naturally favor certainty, the status quo. It's a far more comfortable, safe place to be. Discovering that we fall short in some way brings the same response as the Pharisees when Jesus pointed out the error of their ways: pushback, resistance, anger, frustration all stemming from cognitive dissonance—the disturbing evidence that we are not the whole, spiritual, exemplary people we thought we were.

COGNITIVE DISSONANCE

Why is it so hard to believe that we don't have it all together? The failures of the Pharisees and teachers of the law seem so obvious to us. Why didn't they "get it"?

What was wrong with them? Probably the same thing that is wrong with us whenever we discover a failure in our own lives—or worse, when someone else points out a failure in us. The admission that we don't have it all together requires one essential virtue: humility. To admit we are flawed, broken, incomplete, and in need contradicts our carefully crafted personas of "good Christian," which, when properly groomed, even hides the hypocrite factor from our own self-awareness. Thus, pride protects us from facing our real selves.

Therefore God deems it necessary to disrupt our comfort in order to build a more robust faith that helps us to see our weak (sinful) spots, to confess them as failures, and to resolve to walk in truth—in other words, to become more like his Son. That discomfort is *cognitive dissonance* and it is a powerful concept in human development and in spiritual growth.

Saul McLeod defines the concept:

Cognitive dissonance refers to a situation involving conflicting attitudes, beliefs or behaviors. This produces a feeling of mental discomfort leading to an
alteration in one of the attitudes, beliefs or behaviors to reduce the discomfort
and restore balance. Since nearly all of us like harmony in our thinking and
doing, we are disturbed by cognitive disharmony. The disturbance prompts
change in an attempt to restore harmony.[1]

While speculation (chapter six)—thinking about how to use new
knowledge—is driven by reason and emotion, often it has another antecedent:
cognitive dissonance. The term was coined in 1957 by Leon Festinger, a MIT
social psychologist. The concept has been utilized by many others using
similar but different words.[2] It is virtually inconceivable that any significant
human change could be described without using the concept. We will try to
show its use in Scripture and Jesus' own use of it, rather frequently. That suggests we should pay attention to it for our own teaching.

First, here is an example of dissonance in attitudes, beliefs, and behavior:

My attitude: I have anger toward another person, but I have a right to be angry
because of what they did.

My belief: I believe in forgiveness since Christ has forgiven me, but my pain
keeps me from letting go of my resentment toward the other person.

Behavior: Next Sunday I hear the sermon on prayer from Mark 11:25 including
the words: "And when you stand praying, if you hold anything against anyone,
forgive them, so that your Father in heaven may forgive you your sins."

Notice the sequence toward dissonance: anger is a sin, but it can be ratio-
nalized as "righteous anger" (no dissonance). Or, one can forgive; but it
would mean I can no longer hold anger against the offender (potential dissonance). I want to be forgiven by my heavenly Father, so now I am in a bind
(dissonance). My seething anger can continue but then I would be disobe-
dient (more dissonance). That would also make me a hypocrite (serious dissonance). Or, I can forgive the other person, set myself free from the anger,
and enjoy fellowship with my Father (resolution, elimination of dissonance,
and restoration of harmony).

Only when attitudes, beliefs, and behaviors are in alignment with the
values of Scripture can there be peace in our souls. Having the right attitude,

belief, and behavior often tests us severely, but there are no options if god-liness is the goal. Cognitive dissonance is a gift from God to be used by the Holy Spirit to grow us.

THE RESULT OF DISSONANCE

Dissonance usually appears when we have unfulfilled expectations. Think about it. The last time you were frustrated, angry, or disturbed, was it because you experienced an unfulfilled expectation? What were you expecting? What actually happened? If what happened was not what you had hoped for, you probably experienced frustration and perhaps other negative emotions. These are the perplexing moments of cognitive dissonance. Contrary to our wish, answers often elude us and challenge our belief that the God of heaven always does right. In life's disruptive and confusing moments, we must rest in the fact that our loving heavenly Father makes no mistakes.

But most of our dissonant moments are smaller disturbances, like a flat tire at an inopportune time, someone late for an appointment, a promise broken, losing electricity in a storm, and so on. Are all of these just incidents, or is God present with purpose for that stressful moment? We think the latter. He is always about growing our patience; helping us see things more clearly; teaching us not to judge so quickly, to find his peace in troubled times, to feel contentment in the midst of turmoil, to be gentle when impulse says "strike out," to forgive when we think we deserve to be angry, and ultimately, to grow our faith in the trustworthy heavenly Father.

Dissonance also appears when we are confronted with an idea that runs counter to everything we have always thought—when our core assumptions are challenged. At that point we have to find a way to reconcile this new idea or content with what we believe. This is where dissonance takes us on a journey to one of four responses: (1) adopt a new assumption about what is true, (2) adjust it in some way, (3) reject it altogether, or (4) confirm what we believe. Dissonance is a major stimulus for further learning . . . *if* we are open to learning.

THE GOD WHO DISTURBS

We prefer to think of God as the peace giver, comforter, and refuge where nothing disquieting can enter. And he is—but not always. Yet there is always a higher purpose for all God brings our way.

Oddly, the Pharisees did not feel any dissonance about the cavernous gap between their teaching and living—or they didn't care![3] This prompted Jesus to use highly provocative metaphors and disturbingly personal statements when confronting them (e.g., blind fools, whitewashed tombs, snakes, etc., see Mt 23:13-33). Ironically, John the Baptist saw the problem with the Pharisees early on, calling them a "brood of vipers" and admonishing them to "produce fruit in keeping with repentance" (Mt 3:7-8). Still, they resisted.

Perhaps later they repented. That would have been Jesus' primary purpose for such a performance: to help the Pharisees see themselves as he saw them and to immediately bow, confessing their sin and changing their ways so that their teaching and their practices were more congruent with who Jesus was and who Jesus wanted them to be. Thus, Jesus' confrontation with the Pharisees was an act of love—a stern rebuke to be sure, but an act of love from a caring, compassionate Savior who sometimes uses extreme measures to draw people back to himself. Don't you love a Jesus like that?

Much of the dissonance we experience causes us to grow in our faith, a point made above. The Pharisees and teachers of the law were missing the mark by a wide margin. In fact, they fought any change not because their theology was bad but because their life was a contradiction of their teaching, confusing and misleading the people. On one point, however, their basic beliefs and assumptions about Jesus not being the Messiah were wrong, and unless they changed, they would not enter his life (Mt 23:13; Jn 3:16-18). We must always be ready to look deeply into our beliefs and assumptions to make sure they align with the Scripture. Read on.

ENDURING COGNITIVE DISSONANCE

Periods of dissonance; not knowing; living in the fog, darkness, confusion, and uncertainty are called times of faith—walking by faith. Sometimes the purpose for these troubling times becomes apparent in a matter of days, weeks, months. But it may even be years before we see what God was doing and has done. Eventually, when the light of God's own perspective enters our mind, and we see more clearly that he was present and active all through the darkness and confusion, praise begins to resonate through us.

Yes, we do not understand everything in this life and will not until we see with our heavenly eyes. Then, all will be totally coherent, fully understandable, and entirely consistent with God's purposes for us in this earthly life. "For now we see in a mirror, darkly; but then face to face: now I know in part; but then shall I know fully even as also I was also fully known" (1 Cor 13:12-13 ASV). Admission of limited vision should be followed with a humble confession that at best we are unworthy servants with poor vision. Such an attitude will help us minimize the hypocrite factor so insidious and counter to the kingdom.

JESUS, DISSONANCE, AND THE BRAIN

Several studies using the fMRI discovered that when a person experienced dissonance, a conflict between two incompatible options, it showed up in the activated amygdala (emotion). Another region of the brain (a part of the prefrontal cortex), which is associated with control, also became active. It functions to restore a sense of well-being or equilibrium, bringing a sense of satisfaction to the individual that life is back on "track." "Resolving dissonance may help prevent us from making bad choices or motivate us to make good ones," says Keise Izuma, lecturer in the department of psychology, University of York, England.[4]

Let's go back to the Pharisees, the religious leaders enjoying their role as the high-status power people in Jesus' time. As one would expect, they fully intended to keep their privileged positions in the synagogue and society. The presence of Jesus threatened everything they had built and celebrated. Their days were filled with dissonance largely because of Jesus' presence and teaching. Early on they tried to figure out if he was the true Messiah. But if he was, what would that mean for them? Both Jesus' teaching and life presented the Pharisees with a choice: change or try to discredit his claims. As their anger toward Jesus grew, it surfaced yet another dilemma: if they moved against him, the Jewish people would turn against them because the Jews believed Jesus to be the Messiah. This of course brought more dissonance: How could they get rid of Jesus while not risking their lives and reputation? So they rigged a betrayal, held a mock trial, and eventually incited the people to spare the murderer, Barabbas, and crucify Jesus.

Dissonance is about making choices. The Pharisees consistently chose wrong.

Given the powerful claim that dissonance drives human development, another name for what Christians would call Christian maturing, what evidence exists (besides Mt 23) that the Bible condones or even encourages such an idea? That is, can the concept of dissonance contribute to spiritual growth? If so, how does one utilize such a concept wisely and within the constraints of ethics and the working of the Holy Spirit?

If you are wondering how all of this fits into *speculation*, (a dissonance arising in the reader, at this time, perhaps), we are getting there. Dissonance refers to those disquieting life situations whereby we have opportunity to:

- recall what we have learned in order to
- reflect on its value for the disquieting situation so that
- we might speculate on the best/right way to proceed and
- be aware of barriers that might obstruct my decision to act and
- begin to act on my decision with the intention that I might
- form new habits that will lead me to a more coherent, integral life (character)
- culminating in Christlikeness.[5]

As you probably noticed, these points take us through the Learning Cycle with the latter points to be addressed in the following chapters.

In the classroom, the very act of posing open-ended questions often produces dissonance for some learners who prefer just getting the correct answer from the expert. Hearing alternative opinions forces thought, evaluation, and response, which (for some) causes an uncomfortable ambiguity—not being sure of the right answer to memorize. Jesus was not afraid of dissonance; nor should we be. The concept has life-changing implications, and when we understand it more fully, it may open the doors for new interpretations of life situations, especially the difficult ones, and new growth—all of which we want to embrace in our classrooms, homes, churches, and study groups.

JESUS AND HIS DISTURBING TEACHING

A few years ago I read through the four Gospels focusing especially on Jesus' teaching and interactions. What surprised me was the frequency with which Jesus words disturbed the status quo. Sometimes we don't see the contrarian nature of Jesus' words because we have become so accustomed to reading them—or because it is hard to conceive of how it must have disturbed the listeners at that time. But read through the eyes of the people listening, especially the scribes, Pharisees, and teachers of the law—Jesus' contemporary religious leaders and theologians.

The Old Testament Scripture, at that time, rested in the hands of experts. They knew the right answers, and everyone trusted their teachings, including their teaching on the way to eternal life. Anyone contradicting these religious leaders would be accused of blasphemy, a crime punishable by death in some situations. Jesus knew this and still he chose to disrupt their neatly arranged, self-serving religious system. And he does it relatively early in his public ministry. Few speeches in history were more unsettling than the Sermon on the Mount (Mt 5–7).

Virtually everything Jesus pronounced undercut established teaching and practices of the religious elite. Consider the following statements:

- Blessed are the poor in spirit. (Mt 5:3)

- Blessed are those who are persecuted. (Mt 5:10)

- Unless your righteousness surpasses that of the Pharisees and the teachers of the law, you will certainly not enter the kingdom of heaven. (Mt 5:20)

- "You shall not murder. . . ." But I tell you that anyone who is angry with a brother or sister will be subject to judgment. (Mt 5:21-22)

- You have heard that it was said, "You shall not commit adultery." But I tell you that anyone who looks at a woman lustfully has already committed adultery with her in his heart. (Mt 5:27-28)

- You have heard that it was said, "Eye for eye, and tooth for tooth." But I tell you, do not resist an evil person. If anyone slaps you on the right cheek, turn to them the other cheek also. (Mt 5:38-39)

- You have heard that it was said, "Love your neighbor and hate your enemy." But I tell you, love your enemies and pray for those who persecute you. (Mt 5:43-44)

When Jesus said, "You have heard that it was said . . ." he was specifically referring to the teaching of the Pharisees and teachers of the law—openly, bluntly contradicting them. Everyone realized this instantly. They were astonished at the authority with which he spoke and, perhaps, more astonished that he challenged the powerful religious establishment.

Everyone should have been experiencing cognitive dissonance. The religious leaders dug in their heels resisting truth, resisting change. Their response was opposite that of the people who embraced truth, thus embracing Jesus (Mt 7:24-26; 8:1). Meanwhile the teachers of the law and Pharisees began to undermine his authority and plot against him (Mt 9:3; 34).

Matthew 6 contains more shocking contrasts to prevailing religious practices of the day. Jesus explains how *not* to do good (to be seen by others)—rather, do it quietly without pretense; how *not* to pray (standing in public and praying loudly)—rather, pray in private, in your room without display. Fast in a way that no one can tell what you have been doing; don't store up treasures on earth; don't worry about what you will eat, drink, or wear; unlike the pagans, whose priorities are warped, seek first the kingdom of God and his righteousness and the other things will take care of themselves.

Matthew 7 addresses topics like not judging others; beams in the eye; pigs and dogs; a summary of the Law and Prophets ("do unto others"); destiny (narrow and wide gate); false prophets; and as a closing to the sermon, presents a homily on the wise person building on a rock versus the foolish person building on the sand.

Even at the end of his life, Jesus was shattering people's expectations and replacing them with images of who he was and what we should be like. He portrayed leadership as one who serves with unfabricated humility. The last shall be first and the least will be the greatest. Take the lowest seat and avoid the allure of honor. Seek godly character over the façade of titles; resist hierarchy if it interferes with being brothers. Exaltation is bestowed by others and not self-awarded (Mt 23:1-12). For years the people had been accepting the teaching of the Pharisees. To disrupt and maybe dislodge these misguided teachings, Jesus used statements that pushed people to think, to be disturbed, to figure out who was right—who spoke truth. Ultimately at stake was the question, "Is this Jesus the Messiah?" "Is he the One we should worship?" or, in the language of this chapter, "What should I do if Jesus is the Messiah?"

So here is the point: our situation resembles that of the early Jews facing a decision about Jesus. If Jesus is who he says he is, if God through Scripture and creation speaks truth, what ought we to do? "How then shall we live?" to quote a book title. This, of course, is *speculation*, as we saw in this chapter and the last. When we *speculate* about the "So what should I do in light of truth?" our answer must reflect something of the character of Jesus Christ.

ILLUSTRATING DISSONANCE

Muriel and I started dating in Bible school. She was a missionary kid ("MK"), and though I was concerned about missions, I was not drawn to it as a career. She was sensing God was still drawing us together, and she accepted my thoughts. Eventually we married and toward the end of graduate school, I looked for a teaching position. Some positions that opened up were in areas for which I had little interest. The door seemed closed. Entering a PhD program seemed premature with the little experience I had. That door seemed closed too. What to do? The dissonance of not knowing "what next" was emotionally taxing for me.

"They are looking for a short-term missionary to teach in a Bible college in Africa," injected my wife after reading a mission bulletin. "And you can teach in English," she continued. I wasn't expecting that turn of events. *Why didn't God just open up something stateside? That would have been much easier for everyone . . . especially me.* Of course, this news produced even more dissonance. After all, missions had been eliminated from my future (a deeply held belief). For Muriel, however, it meant the possibility of returning to Africa, her childhood home.

After debating with God for a while, mostly telling him why this wasn't a good idea, I began to speculate about what teaching in Africa might be like. Two years of teaching might be enough to get me a job back in the States or maybe even get me into a PhD program. Besides, my curiosity for exploring more of the world could be satisfied. Furthermore, Muriel's mother would be in a neighboring country. And so my pondering went. With my faith being stretched, we made application and arrived in hot, humid South Africa in December 1969.

We liked it so much we stayed for four years, twice our intended stay.

God often uses dissonance to adjust our own feeble plans and get us back on course with his plan—the best one, but not always the easy or obvious one.

Back in the States, Muriel joined the nursing faculty at a local university while I went to graduate school for my second MA at MSU, which then blended into a PhD program. Halfway through, I was offered a job teaching in a non-formal missionary training program. Really? I thought I had served my missionary time with an honorable discharge. *Let me see: low salary, minimal benefits, no status, and a struggling program. What's not to like?*

Is God messing with my comfort level again? He surely was.

THE REST OF THE STORY

Teaching pre-field missionaries while taking doctoral classes in education was a wonderful blend of theory and experience. I added a cognate area of study in cross-cultural communication, which opened a new world of insights and unexpected opportunities. After seventeen years in missions, twelve of those training pre-field and furloughing missionaries, I looked back. God was so amazing. But in those latter years God was unfolding yet another story preceded by more dissonance (of course).

A business professional working with a telecommunications company in the Middle East had experienced cultural struggles. He and his wife came to our training program and declared, "This is exactly what the multinational corporations need to succeed." Muriel and I combined our skill sets and for the next fifteen years trained personnel from about a dozen Fortune 500 companies. This part-time role in the corporate world, which I enjoyed immensely, became another "mission piece." We helped Christians going out with corporations to locate missionaries and churches in their new country. Now it all fit together. God's plan included the multinational culture as well as the missionary culture. It all made sense. Going to Africa opened a wide door far beyond my dreams.

Next I took a job at a Christian college partly because our two sons could be nearer their grandparents, uncles, aunts, and cousins for the first time in their lives. But then God orchestrated still more dissonance: writing a book. I vowed never to do this because the market was flooded with never-read, little-value books already. The thought gagged me. *I have better things to do.* Then reality hit: if I wanted to stay at this school and get promoted, writing a book was necessary.

More shock (dissonance) arose. For my book to get a favorable hearing depended largely on one person who, for some reason, was not especially fond of our department and who, I found out later, had expressed opposition to my being hired. In fact, she announced to our first faculty department meeting she would be recommending to the board that our department be closed. So it seemed to me that before I even started my job, it was over! Now, working with this same person for promotion gave me shivers. "Haven't I had enough dissonance for one lifetime?" I told God.

But, alas, through a most unusual set of circumstances she liked my book proposal and enthusiastically supported its publication. *Cross-Cultural Conflict* has been reprinted nearly every year for the past twenty-six years. People actually were reading my book . . . lots of people. A few years later, for my tenure, I wrote *Cross-Cultural Connections* and later *Cross-Cultural Servanthood* (all

InterVarsity Press) with combined sales of about 150,000 copies. Add to that consulting, traveling, and ministering in about a hundred countries and concluding our careers teaching in a PhD program at a great school. Never in my wildest dreams could I have envisioned such a future. God's stunning generosity continually amazes me. I am eternally grateful that God disrupted my plans for his own. I am deeply humbled that he would allow me to partake of life with wonderful colleagues, outstanding students, loyal friends, and an astounding family—all of which I am unworthy. Thank you, gracious Father.

WRITE YOUR STORY

When other people tell their stories, they sound so "fairy tale"; everything goes so smoothly, and all works out perfectly. Success comes easily; failure, if at all, is brief. Doubt never occurred to anyone (or so they would have us believe). Faith never wavers and conquers every foe. Frankly, I'm suspicious of those stories—maybe because my story is so messy, filled with bumps, failures, doubt, anxiety, and no little dissonance. It is totally a God story, of his grace, patience, mercy, and forgiveness extended to a country kid coming to faith as an early teen with small ambitions except for one feature: a desire to follow God wherever he led. The good things that happened were wonderful surprises for someone like me, undeserving but steadfast in seeking to follow Jesus and honor the God of my salvation.

Be ready for messiness. When you resolve to follow Jesus and establish new patterns of behavior, expect challenges. Handling those challenges (dissonance) and speculating about how God proposes to use your life is what this chapter and those following are about. Always remember, God's vision of the future is much better than yours.

BACK TO LOVE, COURTSHIP, AND MISERY

In the previous chapter we introduced speculation. In a section called "Love, Courtship, and Misery," I related the story of high school juniors visualizing the probability that they might have a broken marriage (divorce), an unhappy marriage, or a happy marriage. The odds heavily favored an unhappy or broken marriage. One girl wrote that as a result of this learning activity, she had decided not to elope with her boyfriend. Now for the back story.

I learned later that this same girl had an older sister who had eloped a year earlier and was presently going through a bitter divorce. Given this, her decision is even more shocking. Not long after that revelation, I learned that her parents had a very unhappy marriage and were in the process of divorcing. This girl sitting in my Sunday school class was enduring a world of trauma and dissonance. At first, she speculated that her best escape was to elope with her boyfriend. Now, having this experience in the class, she ditches that idea as unlikely to give her happiness. In other words, she re-speculates after considering her decision. While she cannot yet figure out the way forward, she knows it is not eloping—a wise decision, for sure. And I believe it was the power of this learning task (a simple simulation) that caused her to hear God's voice not to elope. Reading her words, "As a result of this class I have decided not to elope with my boyfriend," brought an impulse to pray for God's grace and wisdom to continue guiding her.

Speculation is when we make choices. Those choices, sometimes hard choices, made with the guidance of the Holy Spirit and the steadfast commitment to do the will of the Father, do not come with promises of ease, fame, and fortune but do come with God's promise that "I am with you always" (Mt 28:20) . . . "never will I leave you . . . [nor] forsake you" (Heb. 13:5-6; see also Gen 28:15; Deut 31:6; 1 Sam 12: 22; 1 Kings 8:57; Ps 73:23-26; Is 41:9-10). We pray that, as you write your story, these verses will anchor you in the troublesome, dissonant times and always keep you in the path of obedience as you marvel in God's love, grace, and wisdom.

SUMMARY

Cognitive dissonance, a piece of life most of us prefer to avoid, can actually be a gift from our loving Father who seeks our growth and well-being. Seeing disruptions as times in which the Holy Spirit is active in building Christlike attributes in us strengthens our faith and builds our character. Dissonance, managed from a faith framework, creates whole people who are more functional as kingdom builders doing all to the honor and glory of Christ.

Barriers to Change

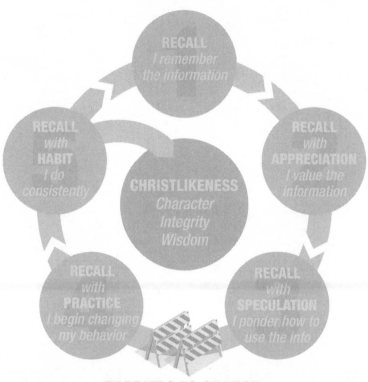

BARRIERS TO CHANGE

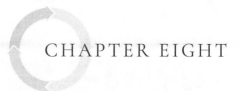

CHAPTER EIGHT

Identifying Barriers

Consider it pure joy, my brothers and sisters, whenever you face trials of many kinds, because you know that the testing of your faith produces perseverance.

JAMES 1:2-3

If you think you can or, you think you can't, you are right.

HENRY FORD

OW MANY TIMES have you come to a new year and decided that this coming year, things are going to be different? It is almost a joke as the new year rolls around: How many days it will take before we fall flat on our faces and toss the resolutions? Five days? Ten days? A month? Four months? In fact, researchers have enough data now to predict how long. According to a December 2015 article in the *U.S. News & World Report*, 80 percent of us tend to abandon our New Year's resolutions by Valentine's Day.[1] The article continues, "it's important to recognize that (resolutions) . . . are doomed to fail if . . . you've done nothing to enhance your capacity to either sustain motivation or handle the inevitable stress and discomfort involved in change. . . . '[I]t's not the horse that draws the cart, it's the oats.'"[2]

Strategic thinking about managing the stress and barriers to change is key to success. When I (Muriel)[3] begin to falter in keeping a resolution, I tend to redouble my efforts and carry on for a while longer.

But eventually, most of us see our best intentions evaporate. When God calls us to make important life changes, failure can be especially critical. The consequences can be even more critical. Satan especially is not happy when he sees any of us decide to live a more authentic, Biblical life. He is the great adversary. In John's Gospel, Jesus calls him a "liar" and "the father of lies" (Jn 8:44). Satan loves to see us try then fail to obey God's commands because of the difficulties. Paul warns us in Ephesians 6:12, "For our struggle is not against flesh and blood, but against rulers, . . . against the powers of this dark world and against the spiritual forces of evil in the heavenly realms." Satan sets up various blockades to deter and confuse us. We need God's power to overcome his lies. Unfortunately, however, Satan often needs to do nothing at all. Our own bad habits sabotage us. In ways we did not expect, hurdles block our way, dashing our hopes for change.

This chapter addresses those barriers we will likely encounter whenever we try to act upon what we learn and what we are convinced we should do. We can identify some of the barriers ahead of time and make plans to defeat them. We can help our learners do the same. How do we do this? Speculating on what would keep us from acting—even before we act—begins a strategy for success. A second strategy for success is to identify what caused us to fail after our first efforts and to use that failure as a learning tool to success. (See more about this second strategy in the Level IV: Recall with Practice chapters.)

We recognize that throughout the entire Learning Cycle there will be obstacles to impede learning. Many obstacles have already been addressed earlier on in the book. We write about how to avoid learners' loss of attention during a lecture or how to avoid shallow, rote learning by using rehearsal and repetition. We discuss how to challenge learners to speculate on what difference an idea can make in their lives and help them move on toward transformation. We have specifically placed our discussion of barriers here in the Learning Cycle because it is at this juncture between the knowing and the doing that barriers are most likely to hinder or even arrest behavior change or transformation.

A POTENTIAL BARRIER AVERTED

I vividly recall the fear that gripped me as I began to consider embarking on a PhD. In an attempt to avoid that gut fear of failure, I made a suggestion to my mentor, Dr. Ted Ward, "Why don't you just let me take a few courses and see if I can do it?" Ted would have none of that. His encouragement that I was capable, along with Duane's unfailing support, finally led to me submitting the application. I feared what I thought was a major barrier, failing to measure up, and I found their encouragement sufficient to overcome it and move forward. (See more later regarding how the approval of significant others can contribute to overcoming barriers to action.)

Without speculating on potential barriers, we tend to build unrealistic expectations. Then our best intentions fall apart after the first or second speed bump. Failing to make needed changes in light of Scripture afflicts each of us. Knowing the truth but not doing the truth is a dark theme woven through the entire Old and New Testaments. History is loaded with good intentions that vanished into the sands of time. Yet God still calls for repentance and obedience because as our Creator, he knows best how to help us lead meaningful lives.

RECOGNIZING POTENTIAL BARRIERS

Let me begin with a lesson I learned several years ago. While the director of USAID Child Survival programs at World Relief, I found myself in the mountains of Peru spending time with a young Peruvian woman, a health promoter in a remote village. I'll call her Maria. It was obvious from her nonverbals the minute I started talking with her that she was desperately unhappy. I asked what was wrong. She poured out a story that revolutionized my thinking as an educator.

It seems that she had been faithfully teaching the mothers in her neighborhood how to avoid the typical conditions that so often killed the babies and toddlers in her village. One of these deadly worldwide scourges is dehydration from diarrhea. The difficulties of maintaining sanitation and securing clean water causes rampant diarrhea in majority world countries. However, if a mother of a baby with diarrhea is taught the simple practice of continually spooning a mix of clean water and rehydration salts into her child's mouth, most of these temporary episodes can be treated successfully.

A young mother, Juanita, had brought her baby son with diarrhea to Maria the night before. She asked Maria to remind her how to administer the rehydrating fluid. Together they went over the steps of boiling the water, mixing the solution and spooning it gradually into her son's mouth. Juanita went home and followed Maria's instructions all the next day and during the next night. He began to recover.

The next morning, Juanita had to go out to her field, some distance away, for the day. So she turned to her mother, the baby's grandmother, for help. She showed the grandmother exactly what she should be doing for him while she had to be away at her field and then left for the day.

Late that afternoon, she arrived home horrified to find her son close to death. Immediately she took him back to Maria. Maria saw that it was too late. They tried but could not save his life. Now they were getting ready to bury him. When the grandmother was asked what happened, she responded out of her own ancient cultural wisdom. "We all know never to give a child with diarrhea more fluid. It only does more harm than good." I put my arms around Maria and mourned with her and encouraged her. She had done all she could.

It was then we realized our Learning Cycle did not account for those barriers (beliefs of traditional grandmothers, in this instance) people encounter when they begin to follow through on what they learned. Barriers can totally derail the first tentative steps towards doing what is good or best. That grandmother's traditional wisdom kept her from practicing the one thing that could have saved her grandbaby's life. She overruled her daughter's rehydration lesson because her own belief was far better (from her traditional perspective). She was doing her very best for him given the light that she had. Only here the "light" was actually a barrier that resulted in tragedy.

TRADITIONAL WISDOM THAT SUPPORTS THE GOOD

The "wisdom of the people" in a culture, including our culture (often called old wives' tales), can set up major obstacles or barriers to changing behavior. But we cannot always be so quick to judge. Traditional cultural wisdom sometimes supports the good. When working with Khmer mothers in Cambodia, I was delighted to discover it was customary to give rice water, a cereal-based fluid, to a baby with diarrhea.

Simultaneously, new medical research was emerging demonstrating that cereal based fluids helped slow dehydration in babies suffering with diarrhea. Here was a beautiful example of the wisdom of the people that preceded any scientific discovery by decades if not a century or two. In our Cambodian Child Survival program, I made it a point every chance we could to celebrate those grandmothers for their cultural wisdom. This cultural wisdom was an example of God's common grace operating in the minds of those Khmer mothers.

How do we discover barriers to change? A simple set of questions known as a *barrier analysis* helps learners be successful in their attempts to achieve behavior change. There are two steps to any barrier analysis. First, the barriers must be identified. Second, plans are made to overcome, sidestep, or remove those potential barriers.

IDENTIFYING BARRIERS TO CHANGE

What sorts of barriers can and will stymie positive life changes? How can educators equip learners to identify and overcome them? Working to conduct a barrier analysis along with the learners is an important step. Now we turn to a discussion of types of barriers.

A serious discussion with learners about barriers must take place prior to any attempts at change and then again after

> *Insight alone does not necessarily bring about behavior change.*
>
> JAMES O. PROCHASKA, CARLOS C. DI CLEMENTI, AND JOHN C. NORCROSS, "IN SEARCH OF HOW PEOPLE CHANGE"

the first tentative efforts at practicing the new behavior (taking action). Those first attempts at change are precisely where real life takes over from cognitive speculation (Level III) and collides with forces in reality that could derail good intentions. So often, attempts to enact some change in our behavior fails just after the starting gate precisely because a potential obstacle has not been identified, suggesting a plan had not been devised to overcome it.

Identifying possible barriers to change takes careful thought. So much depends on what you hope to change, the level of difficulty involved in that change, the environment where change is to take place, and finally, what you think about when contemplating the change. But be encouraged, it is generally possible, together with the learners, to identify some of the major barriers they will most likely encounter and to create specific plans for overcoming them.

The learners themselves have good insights into their own reality. With guidance, they will identify likely barriers in their own experience. As teachers we can guess what the barriers are, but the learners themselves are the best judge because they know and live in their own reality. And they can design an action plan to overcome those barriers.

The barrier analysis literature has a long history in organizations wanting to avoid failures related to behavior change. The familiar SWOT analysis (strengths, weaknesses, opportunities, threats) approach used by organizations is a type of barrier analysis. More recently, the international health community has developed excellent barrier analysis training manuals. This was done precisely because it is so critical to initiate new behaviors if you hope to promote vibrant health and prevent certain diseases or epidemics. These training manuals depend heavily on gathering data from the people themselves in the community. Community members are most aware of what would keep them from initiating the best health practices.[4]

Jesus identifies barriers to change. Jesus' parable of the sower provides a good starting point for our thinking. In this parable, he identifies the two major types of barriers to learning and growth—personal factors and social pressures—while naming three specific barriers that grow out of those personal and social categories. We find the parable of the sower in three of the four gospels (Mt 13:1-23; Mk 4:1-20; Lk 8:4-15).

Jesus couched much of his teaching in parables, essentially concrete stories, to graphically illustrate abstract truths. He brilliantly used stories to capture the interest of his audience (engagement) and bring the truth home by nestling it down into their daily lives. Using familiar stories to illustrate the truth made what he taught supremely relevant while compelling his hearers to discover the truth for themselves. Discovered truth always requires a much higher level of engagement, which activates and reinforces neural networks within the brain.

All great teaching begins from the here and now, in order to get to the there and then.

WILLIAM BARCLAY,
THE GOSPEL OF MATTHEW

One truth Jesus drives home with this parable is the fact that *hearing* the truth does not always result in *doing* the truth; that is exactly the primary problem we hope to address in this book. Each gospel writer carefully but clearly places the responsibility on every person to respond to the truth.

The hearers' responses vary depending upon the "soil" or heart of each. Almost always, certain barriers stand in the way of doing the truth. Jesus identified three specific barriers or obstacles that explain why people (types of soil) who hear the truth about the kingdom (the seed) fail to let that truth make a difference in their lives (no fruit). In the end, he describes the person (soil) in whom the truth (seed) grows and thrives.

In the story, the first barrier to growth and harvest is seed that falls by the wayside. Birds come along and snatch it up. The soil is hard and well-trodden. This soil represents hearers whose hearts are closed and indifferent to the truth. People with hard hearts never gave the seed of truth a chance to have a place in their hearts and minds. Barclay calls it a shut mind. Consequently, they never invited the truth into their life. The hard soil and shut minds indicate where the Pharisees and teachers of the law found themselves with regard to Jesus and his divinity. They are stuck at the recall level, having heard (cognition) the truth from Jesus about God's kingdom but seeing little value (emotion) in pursuing it. They rejected God's truth at the outset—a personal barrier.

Second, there is the seed that falls on rocky ground with little soil to sustain it. When the sun comes up, scorching the new plants, they wither and die. Rocky ground represents hearers who in the beginning appreciated the truth, saw its value for their lives, but lacked the will or the motivation to sustain obedience once tested by difficulties and persecution (barriers). These hearers made it through the recall, appreciation, and speculation levels but then encountered barriers they were not prepared to confront and gave up trying. Their commitment was not deep enough to withstand social and cultural pressures. Their belief in the value of the truth about Jesus was not strong enough to help them persevere against this pressure from their peers and significant others.

Third, Jesus describes the seed that falls on thorny ground and is choked by the thorns. Again, these hearers initially appreciate and value the truth but then become distracted by other pursuits like "wealth" or "cares" of this world. The thorny-ground hearers may recall the truth of the kingdom, have valued it and even speculated on how to practice it enough to see some growth, but now the barriers loom from within rather than from without. Competing personal ambitions or fears crowd out final integration of truth into practice. The learner isn't sufficiently convinced—doesn't really believe—that the change required is more important than the desires for worldly riches and comfort. Following Jesus, in the end, just isn't worth it to them.

Finally, Jesus tells of the seed that falls on good soil, takes root and produces a good harvest. The hearers integrate the truth of the kingdom into a lifestyle reflecting a character and a daily life honed by God's truth, thus illustrating the successful completion the whole Learning Cycle. These hearers persevere in doing the truth until fruit is evident.

In this simple parable, Jesus captured the core problems we can expect to face when we try to be *doers* of the truth and not simply *hearers* only. Personal forces within us and social forces around us create obstacles to a long, sustainable obedience to truth. Fears about our own capabilities to change, fears about what others will think if we change, and, finally, fears about the costs of change summarize the major barriers learners face when they choose to act on what they are learning. As educators we have a solemn responsibility to create learning tasks that help our learners think hard about what might stop them from practicing the right and the good and to help them then consider how to deal with those barriers.

Do not merely listen to the word, and so deceive yourselves. Do what it says.

JAMES 1:22

Jesus' parable of the sower expressed precisely what social scientists have discovered since then. Research in behavior change identifies three types of barriers: (1) personal—negative thoughts and beliefs about one's capacity to change (my fears), (2) social—negative pressures from significant others leading to no change (fears of others' reactions), and (3) cultural beliefs and practices—pressures from (fear of violating traditional) cultural norms and accepted wisdom that supports the status quo. These can limit how we behave.[5] Clearly social and cultural beliefs and practices can overlap. Once barriers are identified, ways to manage them must be considered. The next section identifies a social science theory that will give us further insight for identifying barriers to behavior change.

THE REASONED ACTION APPROACH (RAA) BEHAVIOR CHANGE THEORY

The Reasoned Action Approach (RAA) theory was developed by Azjen and Fishbein (1975, 1980) to predict the antecedents of behavior change. If we know what tends to cause behavior to change, we can work to create those circumstances that foster it. Initially the focus for RAA was on changing health behaviors. It is also known as the Theory of Planned Behavior (TPB). Data from thousands of studies over the last four decades lend strong validity to this theory. The RAA theory "actually identified a small set of causal factors" for behavior.[6] This social psychological research has since been applied to other fields interested in adjusting behavior, including education.

The core of the Reasoned Action Approach (RAA) theory asserts that a few specific beliefs control both why and when people decide to change their behavior. The stronger the beliefs, the more likely people will achieve their intended behavior change. To change a behavior and for that change to be lasting, people need to be convinced of and to hold these five beliefs:

1. The anticipated behavior change will be beneficial (behavioral belief).

2. Others important to them will approve of the behavior (normative/ social belief).

3. They are personally capable of changing the behavior (control/personal belief).

4. They have some control over what would help them perform the behavior (control/personal belief).

5. They also have some control over what would hinder their ability to perform the behavior (control/personal belief).[7]

Consequently, how we teach and the learning tasks we create for the learners can influence the strength of their beliefs, which then tend to influence potential new behavior.

To pursue a certain action, people should carefully consider whether or not they can answer the following five questions based on the five beliefs above. As you ask the following questions of your learners, you could suggest they answer in writing using a Likert scale of 1 to 3 to indicate how strongly they believe it: 1 = weak belief, 2 = moderately strong belief, 3 = strong belief. This learning task points to where they might need do more thinking.

1. How much do I believe that the new behavior is beneficial and worth my pursuing?

2. Do I believe with confidence that important people in my life will approve of my doing this new behavior? (Or, does it matter to me if they approve?)

3. How strongly do I believe I have the capability to do this new behavior?

4. Do I have a realistic perspective of what barriers I will encounter as I change my behavior, and can I control those hindrances?

5. Do I have a realistic perspective of what supports will help me to change my behavior, and can I control those supports?

Remember the story of the grandmother earlier in this chapter who did not give her grandson the fluid he needed to survive an episode of diarrhea? She was gripped by a strong traditional belief that contradicted her daughter's new belief (need for fluids). She doubted (the RAA theory belief one above), that administering fluids would benefit the boy although Juanita, the boy's mother, strongly believed in his need for fluids.

Then, sadly, Juanita did not take into account her mother's lack of approval and falsely assumed that her mother would carry through with the new way of preventing dehydration and the death of her son. That miscalculation (related to belief two) resulted in tragedy.

When I considered pursuing a PhD, I initially doubted belief three above. I was not sure I was capable of doing the work. I needed both Duane's and Ted's assurance that I was indeed capable. These initial doubts often limit us from even beginning to change.

Then our new year's resolutions often fail because we have not planned to deal with potential difficulties we face (belief four) or we have not taken advantage of what could support our efforts to change our behavior (belief five). For example, do I have the encouragement of people important to me to pursue the behavior?

As teachers we know we cannot compel anyone to believe something. But we do have the responsibility to engage the learner in thinking about each of these questions and to be realistic about the barriers they will encounter in the process. Beliefs can be strengthened when they are brought to the learners' attention, considered, and discussed. You may ask, how do these beliefs fit into the Learning Cycle?

The Reasoned Action Approach and the Learning Cycle. Although the beliefs identified in the RAA research cannot be precisely correlated with each level of the Learning Cycle level, it is helpful to highlight where a specific belief tends to develop at each level of the cycle. The first belief that the new behavior is worth pursuing fits best into the first two levels of the Learning Cycle: Recall "I remember the information" and Recall and Appreciation "I value the information." The overarching learning goals in these first two levels are to (1) consider new content/ideas/truths—the truth is worth my knowing (Level I: Recall) and (2) identify the importance of the content—its power to change one's life for good—and value that change enough to pursue it (Level II: Recall with Appreciation).

The second and third RAA critical beliefs, "Will others approve of my doing this?" and, "Am I capable of integrating new behavior into my life?" will tend to be answered in the third Learning Cycle level (Recall with Speculation) and in conducting a barrier analysis. At this level the learning goals are to (1) imagine (Recall with Speculation) what one might achieve, accomplish, or both, and (2) believe I have a realistic perspective on what will hinder me (barriers) and what will help me (ways to overcome the hindrances) as I begin to practice the new behavior.

Most relevant to our barriers discussion are the two beliefs surrounding the questions, "What will others think about my new behavior?" (normative or social beliefs) and, "What do I think I will realistically face to help or hinder me when I try to take action?" (personal control beliefs). Fears about how others will react to new behaviors or fears about one's own capacity to sustain a new behavior is often so daunting that we don't decide to act. On the positive side, knowing what beliefs need to be strengthened can help these beliefs become powerful tools to stay on track when initiating a new behavior.

Because sustainable habits, or routines, are such potent means for overcoming barriers to change, we deal with habit formation in much

> *Even as you read these words, a tiny portion of your brain is physically changing. New connections are being sprouted—a circuit that will create a stab of recognition if you encounter the words again.*
>
> GEORGE JOHNSON, *IN THE PALACES OF MEMORY*

greater depth when we get to Level V: Recall with Habit. In this chapter we (1) identify relevant barriers to a behavior change and (2) build a realistic plan to address them even before they are encountered. How then do we go about this barrier analysis?

A barrier analysis illustration. A couple of years ago, I assisted a global church-based relief and development agency in developing a week-long curriculum. The goal was to teach African pastors and church leaders some basic biblical passages on the church's responsibility to reach out and help the vulnerable in their community. We tested our draft of the curriculum in Malawi

by asking African leaders to teach the entire one-week curriculum twice. The
week-long curriculum was specifically designed to help church leaders with
God's help to take new action in six specific areas of desired behavior:

1. Commit his/her own life to Christ.

2. Never depend on a traditional healer (witchdoctor) again, but rather,
   trust in God.

3. Teach another person about a harmful (cultural) belief and replace it
   with God's truth.

4. Take steps to restore a broken relationship in his/her life.

5. Join or form a group in church to help people in need.

6. Take one action to reach out to a neighbor in need.

At the end of the teaching week we conducted a barrier analysis to help us
revise the next draft of the curriculum. To do this we held focus groups with
all who had just experienced the teaching related to the six desired behaviors
in the curriculum. For desired behavior three, several harmful but commonly
accepted cultural beliefs had been addressed during the week and how God's
truth replaces that lie. One of those harmful beliefs was that only boys, not
girls, should go to school.

We asked the church leaders who had just received the training questions
such as, "What would prevent other church leaders from telling someone that
their belief is harmful?" Several answers were revealing.

"Some church leaders also believe those lies, so they have no authority to share."

"We are afraid members will leave the church."

"Cowardice or being afraid."

Each of these three answers relate to personal or social norm beliefs that
need to be countered. Simple barrier analysis questions like these will invariably spark thoughtful discussion with the learners about how to counter
obstacles that might interfere with taking the desired action. Remember, the
learners themselves are generally best able to identify particular barriers
within their own life context.

We also asked the church leaders in their focus groups, "What would keep
a church member from helping a vulnerable person in need?"

"They know they will get nothing from the needy."

"They look down on the needy."

"Sometimes they don't think they have enough to share."

All three answers reveal barriers that grow out of personal beliefs and fears church members may have. The first two answers point to a need for more teaching. We needed to revise the curriculum to emphasize the image of God within every human being and God's compassion for every human being. Answers from the focus groups yielded insights into the thinking of the Malawian church leaders and the problems they expected to face in their churches. It also generated some solid information on barriers needing to be addressed in the curriculum revision.

Learning task: barrier analysis questions. The following template can be used with virtually any group to identify barriers to any goal they wish to achieve. As illustrated above, we used it with Malawian pastors and church leaders, but you can ask these questions in any cultural context of children, community groups, Bible study group members, or students in any classroom in public, baccalaureate, or graduate school.

Simple questions to elicit potential barriers from the learners may take several forms. For example, you could ask,

- "What would make it difficult for you to (insert new behavior)?"

Or,

- "Who might prevent you from initiating or persisting in (insert new behavior)?"

If the learners identify several barriers to changing one behavior, suggest that they prioritize the barriers and think of a plan to counter each one. Sometimes the learners may fear the consequences of the desired new behavior on their relationships. If the learner fears disapproval from others, you might ask,

- "Who would disapprove of your (insert new behavior)?"

Or,

- "Why would they and how would they disapprove of your (insert the new behavior)?"

Once they name the barrier, they can begin to make a plan to counter, minimize, or remove it. As you work with these core questions, develop your own or make modifications as best suits your situation. We see no limits as to where they can be useful. In the next chapter, we explore how to assist learners develop plans for overcoming the barriers they will encounter in their efforts to change behavior.

CHAPTER NINE

Overcoming Barriers

*You, dear children, are from God and have overcome them, because the
one who is in you is greater than the one who is in the world.*

1 JOHN 4:4

*The passion for stretching yourself and sticking to it, even (or especially) when it's
not going well, is the hallmark of the Growth mindset. This is the mindset that
allows people to thrive during some of the most challenging times in their lives.*

CAROL DWECK, *MINDSET*

ONCE PEOPLE BEGIN to practice a new behavior, they invariably encounter barriers they had not anticipated, nor were they prepared
to confront. Once more they need to return to the question, How
do I overcome these new barriers? Teachers and co-learners should expect
to support each other throughout the very awkward, tentative attempts at
behavior change—the application or practice phase (Level IV: Recall with
Practice). Re-cycling regularly into the learners' lives and inquiring how it is
going not only encourages motivation and persistence but also underscores
the importance of what they are trying to do.

HELPING A LEARNER OVERCOME A BARRIER—ILLUSTRATED
A few years ago in Puebla, Mexico, Duane was teaching a group of North
American college students about how to build trust with others, how trust is

broken, and how to begin rebuilding trust—a critical relational skill for cross-cultural success or success in any relationship. One of the young men in the class, Greg, spoke to Duane after the session about how the Holy Spirit had convicted him that he had broken trust with his father. He wondered how he might begin rebuilding that trust. Duane asked Greg to tell him about his father. Greg talked about how good his father was with his hands, making things from wood. "He is really good and loves to work with all kinds of wood," said Greg.

Duane then asked, "Have you seen any unusual pieces of wood around here that your father might like?"

"Actually, I have," Greg responded quickly. Duane went on to suggest perhaps he could mail his dad a piece of wood his father might like and so begin to rebuild some trust. Greg agreed that his father would probably appreciate that gift.

We wish we knew the end of this story, but it was clear this young man needed some help thinking through a plan to rebuild trust with his father. Sometimes a series of open questions posed by the teacher is all it takes for learners to formulate their own plans to overcome some barrier to practicing what the Holy Spirit is nudging them to do.

Planning to Overcome Barriers

Many of the barriers to behavior change grow out of how strongly people believe they can control those factors that either hinder or help them pursue their goal. Consequently, early on, we educators must develop learning tasks to plan for those hindrances. On habit formation, Duhigg writes that those who "never thought ahead about how to deal with" what he called "inflection points" (obstacles) were at a "serious disadvantage" in achieving "willpower habits."[1]

Paul exhorts his readers: "Do not think of yourself more highly than you ought, but rather think of yourself with sober judgment, in accordance with the faith God has distributed to each of you" (Rom 12:3). His call is to humbly and modestly reflect on ourselves—to know ourselves. With honesty we judge our situations, our abilities, our tendencies, and our strengths in light of our faith.

Since opposition is likely from our adversary, Satan, let us be armed and arm our learners. For this reason, we all can pray for discernment; request prayer support from classmates and friends; be aware that Satan will attack;

and be quick to recognize his efforts. John reminds us "for everyone born of God overcomes the world. This is the victory that has overcome the world, even our faith" (1 Jn 5:4). Helping students identify and overcome barriers is a strategy that teachers can employ. Such strategizing is useful within many arenas and hopefully will become a life skill.

Following are a few suggested learning tasks that engage the learners in thinking about their next steps and building skills that overcome barriers.

Learning task: memo to myself. Think back to the Reasoned Action Approach (RAA) theory of behavior change in the last chapter. Research demonstrates that five particular beliefs control the likelihood that people can actually succeed in changing their behavior. The stronger those beliefs, the greater the possibility that a person will succeed in changing behavior. To help learners deepen their commitment to change, the "memo to myself" approach (see chapter three) can be used again, this time addressing two of the five critical beliefs. Ask students to write this memo to myself on the following two topics: (1) the benefits I will experience when I change (a specific behavior), and (2) how I know I am capable of changing (a specific behavior).

Sharing their memos with the teacher or the Bible study leader will further strengthen their belief that they *can* and *should* persevere towards their goal. If they belong to a group of learners working on changing their behavior and there is a high level of trust within the group, it would be appropriate to share their memo with the group. If the group is small (eight or below) each member can share with the whole group. If above eight, break into groups of three to four. Allow for group discussion after each memo is shared. The discussion and affirmation from others will help to confirm and strengthen their original decision. Each time those beliefs are rehearsed and shared, the neural pathway is reinforced and enhances the probability of success. Depending on the situation, you may plan to give some time to prayer within the group.

Learning task: role playing. During my tenure as child survival director for World Relief, the AIDS epidemic began to sweep through our child survival programs in seven countries, killing thousands in its wake. Dr. Gretchen Berggren and I presented this Learning Cycle at an early global AIDS conference in Durban, South Africa. In order to combat the rampant problem of early teen girls being so easily seduced into sexual activity by men and boys, we offered several learning tasks for vulnerable girls. Role playing was but one of those learning tasks.

It was clear that just telling the girls to say, "No!" would likely have little effect the first time they were enticed to have sex with a man or boy. Yet the risks were enormous. It may take only one encounter to contract HIV! Girls, especially teenage girls unaware of the danger of contracting HIV from sexual intercourse, to say nothing of also bearing a child with HIV, must develop the skills to resist such pressures.

Role plays offered a promising approach. It would give them actual practice saying, "No!" and walking away in a simulated classroom context. Several well-planned role plays would offer vivid opportunities to practice resisting in preparation for real life. Physically and verbally going through the motions opposite other young women in the same program would have the added advantage of initiating new neural networks so foundational to creating safe behavior patterns.

If our learning goal is changing beliefs and behaviors, it stands to reason that imaginative role plays designed for defeating barriers can (1) strengthen the belief that success is possible (remember this personal/control belief from reasoned action behavior theory?), (2) identify and highlight barriers learners are likely to encounter, and (3) promote discussion of various ways to counter the feared barrier—whether it grows out of personal fears, peer pressure, or even cultural lies that counter biblical truth.

One of the most elegant uses of role play I can remember was at a conference on conflict resolution. The learning task assigned to us, in groups of four, was: "Describe a conflict you have had with someone in the past, but tell it as though you *are* the other person." To do this we had to take on our opponent's perspective—speaking as our opponent, to say what we thought would have been their argument against us. Spontaneously attempting to see things through an opponent's eyes was a challenging assignment. The debriefing questions after this role play focused on ways to find common ground with our opponents and move toward resolving the conflict.

Think about one of the behaviors you hope to adopt or persuade your learners to adopt. Can you think of a way to use a role play to help strengthen their resolve and familiarize them with the words and actions necessary to counter the obstacle, especially if it grows out of peer pressure?[2]

Learning task: building accountability relationships. Another effective learning task is promoting accountability relationships. Duane does this routinely in his teaching. He gives time in the classroom for learners to commit to an accountability relationship with someone—share their action plan with each other and set a time when they plan to check with each other on how they are following through. If the group schedule doesn't lend itself to creating accountability groups, Duane will assign a learning task by passing out index cards. During a brief period of silence, he encourages them to ask God what changes he is calling them to make, write it down on the card, and add it to their digital calendar. Then, students are to place the card in their Bibles or post it on a bathroom mirror and plan to review the intended change when it comes up in their calendar. Also, he encourages them to ask someone close to them to hold them accountable for that change in the coming days. If learners are willing, Duane asks them to fill out an index card for him, and he will pray for them as well. It is also a good way to follow up with learners. Duane has sometimes shared his own index card with a group.

> *To educate is to guide students on an inner journey toward more truthful ways of seeing and being in the world.*
>
> PARKER PALMER, *THE COURAGE TO TEACH*

Notice here that Duane is using positive social relationships to bolster learners' beliefs that they are capable of their desired change and that someone (or several someones) approves of their making the change. This is where social media could be helpful.

Learning task: managing social pressure. But what about learners who are facing pressure not to change, and the pressure is coming from people who are important to them—their parents, their peers, their spouse, or their employers? These pressures are powerful deterrents to any follow-through. Remember how the research demonstrates that believing people who are important to me (significant others) will approve of the new behavior tends to strengthen the likelihood that efforts to change will succeed? Negative social pressure from those who are important to us can erect enormous barriers to change. Consequently, we must arm our students before they encounter the painful disapproval of others.

- What barriers do I expect to encounter as I begin to change my behavior?

- Who might disapprove of my behavior change?
- How can I respond to their disapproval in ways that don't deter my progress toward my goal?

We need to ask these kinds of questions: "Are there people important to you who will not approve of your choice to change?" "Who are they?" "Why do you think they will disapprove?" "How do you plan to respond to them?" Give your learners time privately to identify them and write out how they plan to respond when the negative comments descend. Sharing these thoughts with a small, empathic group of learners can further expand possible ideas for responding to those who will disapprove. If this social pressure barrier looms particularly large to someone, it might be helpful to do some role playing in order to help them be better prepared for this difficulty.

> *Speaking up is a sign of confidence; being listened to increases that confidence.*
>
> HUGO SLIM AND PAUL THOMPSON,
> *LISTENING FOR A CHANGE*

Always encourage your learners to surround themselves with people who support their chosen new behavior and will provide encouragement and presence in the journey. Positive peer relationships contribute significantly to initiating and sustaining growth.

Learning task: avoiding dangerous contexts. Learners may identify a certain place, a certain person, or a certain group as a major barrier. Exposing themselves to that original situation while they are still in the process of initiating the behavior change could sabotage their good intentions. Alcoholics Anonymous learned this lesson a long time ago. Recovering alcoholics need to stay out of bars and avoid old crowds that love to drink. Drug addicts need to stay away from friends who are users and dealers. Replacing a habit that has negatively influenced one's life means diligently avoiding the context where that destructive habit first took root.

Learning task: managing negative thoughts. Several years after completing my PhD, I was hired to teach several courses at a prestigious baccalaureate college. I had moved from my earlier career teaching nursing into a subject that better fit my graduate work. Before long I began to have panic attacks in the classroom. My new teaching situation was severely threatened. With the help of a counselor, I discovered that I was being sabotaged by my own negative thinking and fear of failing in my new teaching post.

My counselor suggested that before going into the classroom, I write out all my negative thoughts on the left side of a page in my journal. Then, taking those thoughts to God in prayer, one by one, ask him to show me his truth about that thought. I would then write down what I discerned to be God's truth about a particular thought on the opposite side of the paper. It took some time but eventually I began to realize that when I countered my negative thoughts with the truth, I found freedom in teaching once more.

Long held (often false) beliefs about our inadequacies can raise some formidable thought barriers to success. Dealing with those negative thoughts honestly and realistically can go a long way towards overcoming barriers that hinder our progress. The book *Telling Yourself the Truth* is a helpful resource on how to change our thinking.[3]

Occasionally the negativity within a learner is so deep-seated that it raises major barriers to any change—barriers that you, the teacher, perceive will need more help than either you or their peers can offer. Encourage them to seek professional help, perhaps in the counseling service at the institution or from the pastoral staff at a church wherever it might be available in the community.

Learning task: depending on Scripture and prayer. The Scripture lays out God's heart and plans for us. In many passages, God continually calls us to obedience. First John 2:3-4 reads, "We know that we have come to know him if we keep his commands. Whoever says, 'I know him,' but does not do what he commands is a liar, and the truth is not in that person." John 14:21 is clear: "Whoever has my commands and keeps them is the one who loves me. The one who loves me will be loved by my Father, and I too will love them and show myself to them." And finally, in Ephesians 4:1 we read, "As a prisoner for the Lord, then, I urge you to live a life worthy of the calling you have received."

This passage continues in the next two verses with several examples describing that worthy life: "Be completely humble and gentle; be patient, bearing with one another in love. Make every effort to keep the unity of the Spirit through the bond of peace" (Eph 4:2-3). God has promised that if we belong to him, the Holy Spirit within us will lead us into truth and prompt us to act in ways that will honor God. As we obey his word, God uses that obedience to mold us into the person he wants us to be.

The teacher can post a verse a week or email it to class members as reminders of God's presence as they journey into change. Also, they can have students volunteer to post a verse or two that God has used in their journey to stay faithful.

Prayer offers the opportunity to converse with God. As we pour out our thoughts to him, we put our requests before him, ask for the courage to change and ask for wisdom to deal with the barriers. He has promised to answer our requests. We are also encouraged to pray for one another as together we face the barriers to change.

Keep in mind we are still focused on the classroom or your learning context. Satan is unlikely to get disturbed as long as we keep things on the knowledge or cognitive level. It is when we determine to *do* something that causes him to be alarmed and to actively resist our efforts. So expect the battles ahead of us on the road to a more obedient life.

As your students practice that new behavior, we recommend that they memorize this verse: "The one who is in you is greater than the one who is in the world" (1 Jn 4:4). Repeat it several times during the day and especially when the challenge is toughest. As they repeat it, the truth of the verse embeds itself in their memory, strengthening their belief system for the moment and similar moments ahead. Help the learners be prepared ahead of time with a plan to overcome the barriers they expect to encounter.

LEARNING TASK SUMMARY

Prepare learners to overcome potential barriers.

1. Ask the general questions, "What do you hope to change as a result of this truth?" and "What would keep you from doing what you think God is calling you to do?" This question could identify barriers that only the learner could name.

2. Help them set realistic, achievable goals. Success stimulates additional effort.

3. For each goal, ask the learners to identify small, incremental steps toward achieving the goal.

4. Encourage learners to support each other by listening and thinking with classmates on what they expect to encounter as they begin to act on their new thinking. Then pray for them.

5. Ask questions related to how confident they are in their own ability to establish new behaviors.

6. Encourage them to look at past challenges and how they overcame them.

7. Ask questions about what significant others (parents, spouses, bosses, close friends) will think about the changes they are making and how they plan to deal with negative responses.

8. Ask what advantages they have that will help them follow through on their decision to add a new behavior to their lives.

9. Above all, encourage them to persevere even if their first attempts fail.

We have explored how to help learners identify barriers to change and plan to overcome them. In the next chapter we address practicing the new behavior outside the classroom. Learners will still need the support of teachers, Bible study leaders, and peers to realize the transformation.

Recall with Practice

I begin changing my behavior

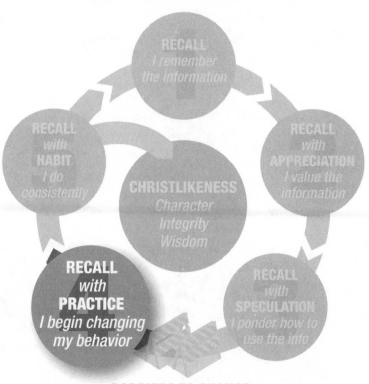

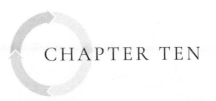

CHAPTER TEN

Transformative Learning

Whatever you have learned or received or heard from me, or seen in me—put it into practice. And the God of peace will be with you.

PHILIPPIANS 4:9

*Tell me what is it you plan to do
with your one wild and precious life?*

MARY OLIVER, "THE SUMMER DAY"

Excellence is not a gift, but a skill that takes practice. We do not act "rightly" because we are "excellent," in fact, we achieve "excellence" by acting "rightly."

PLATO

WE NOW ARRIVE at Level IV: Recall with Practice—"I begin changing my behavior." So far, the learners have encountered a truth (Recall), valued its relevance to their lives (Recall with Appreciation), and then decided to act on that truth by speculating on what actions to take and what barriers may emerge as they begin to put that truth into practice (Recall with Speculation and Barriers). The next step is to do it for the first time (Recall with Practice). They are now "learning-by-practice."[1] Those first attempts always feel awkward and a little risky. Starting a new behavior pattern is always awkward because it is new territory. With a little practice the awkwardness will turn to comfort and eventually to habit.

EARLY ATTEMPTS AT CHANGE ARE UNCOMFORTABLE

Several years ago, we were asked to co-teach a group of pastors in China. The goal was to introduce them to additional teaching methods beyond the lecture. It was a week-long course. When asked by our Chinese host how we planned to approach the course, we responded that since we knew so little about the context these pastors experienced in their teaching, we planned to begin by asking them a series of open questions. As career educators, we knew how easy it is for a teacher to bypass the needs of the learners and ignore their cultural setting. We were also looking for points of relevance we could reference and build upon.

We were unprepared for the fears expressed by our eminent Chinese-American host. He told us that Chinese students do not expect to talk or discuss in the classroom. He also said that to approach the course in that way would suggest to our learners that we were unprepared for class and lacked knowledge of our subject—it just wasn't done in the Chinese setting. We countered by explaining our commitment as educators was to engage our learners in the content, to get them thinking about how they were teaching in their own context.

We could not teach how to get learners engaged if we did not do the same with them. It would be like teaching someone how to swim but never letting them get in the water. We had to practice what we were teaching. We had faced similar situations in several other countries and felt somewhat confident . . . somewhat.

With some trepidation we faced our first day teaching these forty distinguished men and women. We wanted to honor our host by being successful teachers. But we also knew from experience that merely lecturing all week from our own Western perspective would probably be of little value to these pastors. Duane began the course by presenting a couple important educational principles. Then, he asked a couple of open questions about how one of these principles might work in their own teaching experience. He waited for their response. He was met with silence. (Teachers hate silence.)

Explaining a little more, he then ventured another question and we watched their faces. It was obvious from their nonverbals that he was asking them to do something highly unusual. Little by little, Duane continued speaking and then posing another question related to their own teaching experience. Finally, after several attempts at posing questions and what seemed like an eternity to us, an elderly pastor spoke up in response to a question. He briefly talked about a particular experience teaching in the churches where he had responsibility. Duane affirmed him, thanking him for helping us understand his situation. (Later we learned that this pastor was responsible for about twenty-five churches and several thousand church members; he was actually an important leader within the group.) After that, the pastors began to recognize that we really wanted them to think and talk with us. We were elated since we are committed to the truth that the engaged learner always learns more effectively.

They tentatively began responding to our open questions. This new way of engaging content in class with the teacher was not easy for these traditional Chinese. Within a day or so most felt comfortable speaking up. A few pastors never felt comfortable enough to speak during that course but showed they were listening and mentally engaging. We were encouraged. By the end of the week it was clear we had successfully protected our host's reputation and relieved his fears. Many of the pastors were enthusiastically discussing and sharing their perspective on the content to the point where we actually had to begin cutting off discussion. In fact, their evaluations at the close of the week were filled with specific comments about what they had learned and planned to do.

Be prepared for discomfort. We share this illustration because it reminds us of the anxious feelings and fear of failure we had as we began to conduct the course. We remember the intensity of our feelings—how would we engage those pastors, our concern for the reputation of our Chinese host, and the awkward first few hours of class (yes, hours) as our questions plopped flat on the floor in front of us. Those early attempts at behavior change—for us, capturing the attention of the Chinese pastors; for them, beginning to actually engage verbally in the classroom—were fraught with a strange sense of awkwardness.

We have heard from several others who teach in cross-cultural contexts that they have the same experience of silence and hesitation when they ask questions, especially open questions. It isn't that people from other cultures learn better from pure lecture, but that it is typical behavior in their school systems. Once given an opportunity to engage productively in a discussion where they feel safe to speak up, they are generally freed up to think more deeply, and the usual hesitation lessens or disappears. They tend to fully engage with the content and learn from the discussion regardless of cultural restraints. It appears that being engaged and voicing ones' thoughts and questions is universal to effective learning that occurs across cultural differences. It has been our observation that students talk readily outside the classroom; why are they silent as soon as the teacher appears? We found this in Russia too. In most countries we have taught in, we observe the learners actively talking prior to class and after class. Yet, as soon as they enter the door of the classroom, they become silent and tend to remain silent. Why?

We do know those uncertain feelings are to be expected whenever learners attempt a new behavior. If, ahead of time, they set their minds to persevere through those early clumsy attempts and work hard to overcome their fears, successful change is more likely. If our learners understand that failure, temporary failure, is an essential part of learning, it will bolster their decision to keep on trying to achieve their behavior change goal. Acting differently always requires an awkward and sometimes embarrassing period of time when you make those first few attempts at the new behavior.

> *People with a growth mindset "view failure as a sign of effort and as a turn in the road rather than as a measure of inability and the end of the road."*
> PETER BROWN ET AL., *MAKE IT STICK*

Depending on the nature of the transformation people are striving to achieve, they often feel foolish, clumsy, and incompetent. Or they find it harder than they expected. Remember the soils in Jesus' parable?

A point bears repeating: the reason we are comfortable with the traditional way is because it had become habitual. As we continue to practice the new behavior, the awkwardness will eventually give way because the new behavior will start to settle comfortably and become a new habit (see the next chapter). As our mentor Ted Ward often told us, "Everything worth doing, is worth doing poorly . . . the first time." Expect it and push on.

THE POWER OF THE WORD *YET*

Years ago, I served as an instructor in a program for language acquisition techniques. My role was to help learners learn how to produce non-English sounds. Since most were North American English speakers, producing these new sounds presented enormous challenges. Each day the teacher, Dwight Gradin, introduced new methods of language acquisition and, later every day, we instructors drilled them in producing a certain set of non-English sounds. As we watched, many of our learners struggled to reproduce the new sounds without success. It was difficult and discouraging for them. But Dwight would encourage them with these words, "*Never ever* say, 'I can't do this *period*.' *Instead*, always say, 'I can't do this . . . *yet*.'"

Then he'd tell stories of people who sometimes worked months and even years until they were actually able to achieve a particular sound in their language of choice. In fact, I believe it was his wife, Barbara, who actually worked for seven years on one particular sound in the Jeh language of Vietnam before she was able to produce

> *Our brains are designed to find and to construct knowledge from errors.*
>
> JOSHUA R. EYLER, *HOW HUMANS LEARN*

it accurately. I have recycled that lesson many times in my own career when the challenge of doing something new seemed almost insurmountable. I'd remind myself, "I can't do this . . . *yet*; but in time . . . I will!"

The fixed and growth mindsets. In her book *Mindset: How We Can Learn to Fulfill Our Potential,* Carol Dweck describes how learners tend to have one of two mindsets or beliefs about themselves: a "fixed mindset" or a "growth mindset."[2] Those with a fixed mindset think their personal characteristics (e.g., IQ or Intelligence Quotient, or their social skills, or whatever) are fixed once they become adults and they just have to make the best of it. Dweck's research showed that people with a fixed mindset tend to "plateau early and achieve less than their full potential."[3] It "creates an urgency" says Dweck, "to prove yourself over and over."[4]

On the other hand, Dweck reported that those with a growth mindset believe that they can always improve or get better. As a result, these individuals tended to attain greater levels of achievement because they believe "that a person's true potential is unknown (and unknowable); that it's impossible to foresee what can be accomplished with years of passion, toil, and training." She also claims it is possible to move away from a fixed mindset and begin to enjoy a growth mindset.[5]

It is clear that learners' achievements tend to correlate positively with the belief that they have the capacity to improve themselves.[6] Going back to the Reasoned Action Approach (RAA) behavior change theory of Azjen and Fishbein (see previous chapter on barriers), we see similar findings. Remember, their change theory states that when people believe they have the capacity to change a certain behavior, that belief tends to correlate with their success at achieving sustainable behavior change?[7]

What do these findings mean for professors, educators, parents, pastors, or those teaching discipleship classes? We need to remind learners who are struggling in their early attempts to change that their brains are wonderfully flexible and malleable. Neuroscientists call it "plasticity" and it simply means the brain enjoys growing and works in their favor and helps them achieve their goal if they just persevere.[8] It turns out that Dwight's word *yet*—three decades ago—was absolutely key to the growth mindset. "I can't do it . . . *yet*." Embrace it. Encourage your learners to embrace it too.

TIME AND REPETITION PROMOTE HABIT

Practice is the repetition of an action in the service of a purpose or goal. Researchers have studied how long it should take between the first tentative attempts at changing behavior and mastery of that behavior. Data shows that the time to build a new habit exceeds the once accepted twenty-one days, instead being an average of sixty-six days.[9] We write more about this in the next chapter where we deal with habit formation. We know that consistent repetition is a major contributor to forming a strong habit because each repetition strengthens the neural networks that execute an action.[10]

> *The simple fact is that repetition strengthens the connections in the brain.*
>
> ERIC JENSEN, *TEACHING WITH THE BRAIN IN MIND*

DIALOG AND DISCUSSION PROMOTE TRANSFORMATIVE LEARNING

Educational researchers concur that a community of learners who dialogue and discuss together experience more successful transformation of thought and behavior.[11] Slim and Thompson in their book on *Listening for a Change* write that "on a purely individual and psychological level, speaking about a certain situation is often the first step towards addressing it."[12] When people take the initiative to name an issue or problem, a category forms in the brain. The category then becomes a "magnet" for new data. Since the brain loves to solve problems, learners get engaged and grow in their attempts to understand and/or solve a problem. Only then can they begin to think about what actions need to be taken to address the problem. Naming an important part of one's reality creates a mental category that opens the door (a new neural network) whereby new information and thoughtful engagement can begin. It launches the journey from knowing to doing.

Earlier in the book, Duane talked about the image of God. It was an academic category for him at first, but some years later he joined a night ministry. Walking the streets of Chicago with a friend one night, they saw a lady in prostitution. Remember? Duane said, "Is that a prostitute?" to which the friend paused and said, "No! That is a person in prostitution." Duane realized he had been seeing people and judging them according to their vocations, activities, and appearances. This was sinful. God saw them as people, human beings first—people to accept, to love, and to respect. That new category, image of God, brought new awareness, new understanding, and new behaviors consistent with the new truth—mind you, not always perfectly consistent but striving and growing.

Here is one more illustration of the value of discussion from a very different angle. We looked for interesting ways to teach our sons how to arrive at valid conclusions. They usually enjoyed these "games." When they were in junior high school, a new sporty car came out, the Pontiac Fiero. It was novel because the engine was right behind the driver's seat. Our sons started looking for them whenever we were driving around. They soon concluded that Fieros came in two colors: black and red. I knew differently but decided to help them learn. I said, "Let's make that our hypothesis and not jump to a conclusion yet. Let's do more observation and see if we can find support for our hypothesis or not." Soon we saw a white one. New data meant we had to revise our hypothesis to include white. Could we now confidently conclude Fieros come in three colors? After some discussion, we decided it might be wise to make yet more observations. We did. Soon we spotted a rare yellow one. So Fieros came in at least four colors. Several more weeks with no new data allowed for the tentative but quite confident conclusion that Fieros did, indeed, come in only four colors (allowing for custom painting, of course).

What's the point? Several actually. The boys did make some preliminary observations (data gathering) but then made a premature conclusion (beliefs and assumptions). Some discussion prompted looking for further data. When new data surfaced, they had to revise their thinking again and—yet again with even more data (yellow color). Using simple things in their immediate world we tried to encourage responsible decision making. Through dialogue in the family (community discourse), we taught them to diligently gather data, make tentative conclusions while remaining open to new data, be patient, and when all the data is in, analyze and make their conclusion (decision). The more important the decision, the more patience, investigation, and care must be given to avoid a bad conclusion. (Note: Fieros were soon taken off the market, since the engines had a bad habit of catching on fire.)

Dialogue and discussion promote the formation of new categories, new thinking. An important educational theorist, Mezirow underlines the power of discussion and discourse in his theory of transformative learning.

Mezirow's theory of transformative learning. In 1978 Jack Mezirow proposed his adult education theory, which he designated a *transformative* learning theory. He explored how sustained behavior change occurs. His research gained considerable influence in the 1990s and continues to be replicated and validated to this day. He demonstrated that when learners change their perspective (worldview) based on a new disorienting truth (dissonance), they ultimately tend to change their behavior in light of that truth.[13] This is what makes it *transformative.* Mezirow's transformative learning theory affirms our Learning Cycle.

His transformative learning theory can be summarized into four learning stages: (1) the disorienting dilemma, (2) critical assessment of one's assumptions, (3) discourse and dialogue with others to consider changing behavior, and (4) taking action to integrate the new perspective into one's behavior. These four stages, when transacted, result in a fully transformed perspective.

1. A disorienting dilemma. Mezirow found that transformative learning is generally precipitated by what he termed a "disorienting dilemma." Another term for the same phenomenon is "cognitive dissonance" and was discussed earlier in the chapters on Level I: Recall. A disorienting dilemma is any experience that challenges a person's habitual ways of thinking, causing him or her to reexamine a basic assumption or belief about ones' life and the world. A disorienting dilemma can be triggered by any number of experiences such as a life tragedy, a new relationship, a challenging book, a compelling teacher—the list is endless. A disorienting dilemma causes enough conflict and confusion in learners' minds to drive them to reexamine basic assumptions and beliefs about a certain matter. Conversion to Christ is an excellent example. What changes in beliefs and assumptions did you make when you became a follower of Christ? Have any of your beliefs or assumptions been reexamined recently?

If educators are committed to God's truth as expressed in the Scriptures, they ought to be addressing disorienting dilemmas in the thinking of their learners. Life itself is full of disorienting dilemmas that challenge our faith or what we believe to be true. Do we know what disorienting dilemmas our learners are experiencing? Can you suggest how we might discover them?

Today it seems more Christians are having crises of faith (disorienting dilemmas): Does God exist? Did Jesus really rise from the dead? Why doesn't God heal? Is there really a hell? What happens after we die? Will I lose my salvation if I have sex before marriage? Why doesn't God do something about evil? Why do the innocent suffer? And so on.

We believe most disorienting dilemmas tend to arise when learners confront new information. Resolution of the dilemma then expands into the following levels.

2. A critical assessment of one's assumptions. Disorienting dilemmas tend to force us to reexamine our assumptions, our beliefs about what is right and true. In order to change our behavior, we must first reexamine what we assume and believe to be true. Assumptions and beliefs about what is true Mezirow labels as "meaning perspectives." These meaning perspectives (worldview) control how we interpret new experiences, in fact, how we interpret life in general. When transformative learning occurs,[14] our meaning perspectives are changed and ultimately lead to a corollary change in behavior.[15]

When a teacher faithfully relates Scripture to their life problems (relevance), learners will be prompted to struggle

> *A worldview is like an internal map that guides us in navigating reality.*
>
> NANCY PEARCEY, *FINDING TRUTH*

with how they should resolve these problems, these disorienting dilemmas, in light of God's Word.

Wasn't that exactly what Jesus was doing when he challenged his disciples in Matthew 5:27-28 when he said, "You have heard that it was said, 'You shall not commit adultery.' But I tell you that anyone who looks at a woman lustfully has already committed adultery with her in his heart"? He was creating a disorienting dilemma, cognitive dissonance, designed to make his hearers *examine one of their basic assumptions.* So much of Jesus' teaching was intended to lay out new ways of thinking about God's purposes for his children in this world, transforming their perspectives, which then can influence their behavior.

A critical assessment of one's assumptions tends to occur in the Learning Cycle level II—"I value the information" and level III Recall with Speculation— "I ponder how to use the information."

3. *Discourse and dialogue with others as they consider changing their behavior.* Mezirow's third stage of transformative learning requires *discourse* (Mezirow's term) or dialogue with others. Discourse allows learners to discover the discontent others share with the old perspectives (assumptions/worldview). He discovered that belonging to a learning community (characterized by discussion and dialogue) is critical to making the journey from knowing to doing the truth. In other words, learners need like-minded travelers on the journey to help them think critically and build the skills necessary to act on what they consider is right and good.

Talk is engaging. . . . But the one essential condition is that talking should be useful talk. Talk that explains, that questions, that invents new ideas, that motivates.

JAMES E. ZULL, *FROM BRAIN TO MIND*

Together then, in dialogue, learners explore new ways of thinking, acting, and planning to change their behavior. Although, Mezirow found that dialogue does facilitate all of his learning stages, he considers it critical in this third stage.

4. *Taking action to integrate the new perspective into one's behavior.* The final and fourth stage of transformative learning is to take action to integrate the new perspective into learners' lives. This stage also requires discourse—or what may be called a "learning community." Together the learners try new ways of acting (new roles), forge new relationships, and build confidence

through practice. Both stages three and four in Mezirow's theory connect directly with Level IV: Recall with Practice—"I begin changing my behavior" and Level V Recall with Habit—"I do consistently."

Learners need a community of colearners who engage each other as they work through the necessary skills and adjustments required to make major perspective and behavior shifts. By the term "learning community," we suggest the formation of intentional discussion groups in which both teacher and learners participate. The neurological literature highlights the effectiveness of these groups along with the teacher in helping learners move through the transformative learning phases to behavior change. Teachers and all who teach others should make provisions for such supportive learning communities, so effective in facilitating learning.

Qualities of an ideal dialogical community. Mezirow lists the qualities of an ideal dialogical community. As you read through this list, imagine how group discussion could help each learner achieve these goals. He writes that learners need:

1. More accurate and complete information

2. Freedom from coercion and distorting self-deception

3. Openness to alternative points of view; empathy and concern about how others think and feel

4. The ability to weigh evidence and assess arguments objectively

5. Greater awareness of the context of ideas and, more critically, reflectiveness of assumptions, including their own

6. An equal opportunity to participate in the various roles of discourse

7. Willingness to seek understanding . . . until a new perspective, evidence or arguments are encountered and validated through discourse[16]

Theological students and transformative learning. In her excellent qualitative research study with German theological students, Marie-Claire Weinski found strong support for Mezirow's emphasis on dialog and discussion as major contributors to transformative learning. She also found a stark similarity between her transformative learning findings and Mezirow's. The students reported it was critical for them to be "in a learning community and . . . (preferred) learning-within-relationships."[17]

Educators simply cannot abandon learners in their first attempts to practice a new behavior when they are most vulnerable to discouragement and failure.

A healthy community of co-learners who will listen, encourage, problem solve, and even challenge will best support successful perspective and behavior change. If we as educators cannot be part of that learning community, we must be certain that it has been created and is functioning well.

> *Speaking is an act of power, and the act of listening demands respect for the speaker.*
>
> HUGO SLIM AND PAUL THOMPSON,
> *LISTENING FOR A CHANGE*

What of the spiritual dimension? A note of caution here. Because Mezirow is an educational constructivist, he believes that all meaning exists within ourselves as we construct both what we understand of the world and how it should be interpreted from experience. In contrast, given our Christian meaning perspective, we accept by faith that God's revelation in Scripture is a trustworthy guide for interpreting life experience. To repeat ourselves, this is why "Recall" is stated at the beginning of every level in the Learning Cycle. While good learning theories can be helpful, our experience must be framed within God's truth as we know it.

Furthermore, Mezirow makes no mention of the spiritual dimension of reality. As a constructivist, he generally does not think in terms of categories like absolute truth as found in the Bible, a personal relationship with God himself, or the power of the Holy Spirit within to teach us and lead us into truth. These three beliefs, fundamental bulwarks for the Christian educator, are never considered in his work. After his original research was completed, several critiques were raised related to the spiritual dimension. Fortunately, a number of Christian researchers such as Weinski and others have explored transformative learning in people of faith since then and have found that at its core, Mezirow's transformative learning phases remain roughly the same for Christian students. These phases and qualities of discourse, then, are human learning processes that we do well to consider and respect as Christian educators.

Contributing conditions to transformative learning. In Weinski's research, theological students reported that the following conditions contributed to their own transformative learning:

1. Dialog and discussion among students, with instructors and with family and friends

2. Interactive instructional class designs

3. Planned ministry experiences

4. A living relationship with God and a spiritual assessment of experiences

5. Personal support and guidance through counseling or mentoring

6. Modeling (mostly by instructors but also fellow students)[18]

Reread this list and ask yourself, "As a teacher, could I regularly ensure or at least promote these conditions for my learners?" Once they make a decision to

> *People talk to learn.*
>
> DAVID A. SOUSA, *HOW THE BRAIN LEARNS*

begin to practice a new behavior, they will reap enormous benefit if surrounded by a learning community that helps them work through the barriers and firmly grasp their intention to change.

Weinski goes on to describe what the students experienced when they put their new thinking or perspectives into practice:

> All students considered the process of putting the new insights and perspectives into practice . . . a challenge. Almost all . . . experienced difficulties or even fallbacks especially because their transformation was so radical. They also experienced difficulties when they . . . were not sure of support and encouragement . . . (and had) a mixture of negative and positive feelings accompanying this process . . . making this life change happen. (Sometimes) they said, "it was a strange feeling . . . as though they were acting out of character."[19]

Note the importance of support and encouragement and the mixture of negative and positive feelings that can be expected. Replacing unproductive or destructive habits always feels strange until the new behavior becomes habitual.

Both Mezirow and Weinski point out how important a supportive community is to transformation. Many of us can personally attest to being strengthened in our own resolve by watching other believers surmount barriers and bear witness to the worthiness of persevering in the faith. Testimonies—those personal stories of how God has been faithful to fellow believers—do influence and encourage us.

Mezirow's learning stages correspond with the Learning Cycle: from the disorienting dilemma that causes the learners to re-examine their assumptions (Recall) through the feelings that accompany that disequilibrium (Appreciation) to the search for new ways to integrate the new thinking into one's lifestyle

(Speculation, consideration of Barriers and the first attempts to Practice) until the efforts result in new ways of behaving (Habits and Character Formation).

THE PRIESTHOOD OF ALL BELIEVERS IS A LEARNING COMMUNITY

In 1 Peter 2:9, believers constitute "a royal priesthood." Those in the entire church, worldwide, are priests. This truth has two beautiful dimensions: a vertical dimension and a horizontal dimension. The vertical dimension declares that as New Testament priests we now approach God through Christ anytime, anywhere, and under any conditions. No travel to a designated place, no sacrifice, no waiting, no human intermediary. In the Old Testament, priests came only from the tribe of Levi. When people wanted access to God they had to do so at specified times, a specified place and with a specified offering (Lev 1–7). Because Christ is our great high priest, we as believers have no limitations on connecting with our heavenly Father (Heb 4:14-16; see also Rom 5:1-5; 1 Tim 2:5).

The horizontal dimension teaches that the priesthood connects us not only with God on an unrestricted basis but also connects us with other members of the body of Christ. The horizontal dimension has profound implications for families, church, school, and mission.

The Old Testament priest (the Levites) had two functions: the vertical function was to represent the people before God, usually done around temple offerings and sacrifices. This function was replaced by Christ becoming our high priest, an eternal priesthood that demolishes the restrictions of the Aaronic priesthood. The second function of the Old Testament priest was to mediate God and his grace to the other eleven tribes and the world—a horizontal function.

As New Testament believers, we have a similar function: to mediate Christ to one another, to our communities and all of God's creation. We mediate Christ when we accurately and daily represent his character and behavior. We do this as we exercise our spiritual gifts (Rom 12:3-8, Eph 4, 1 Cor 12). We believe this teaching is implicit throughout the New Testament but is quite clear in passages that talk about the connectedness of the body of Christ and the interdependence of the parts of the body (Rom 12; 1 Cor 12; see also Acts 4:32; 15:22).[20]

It is noteworthy that there is no hierarchy in the royal priesthood. We are all contributors—necessary contributors for the body's growth. When New

Testament priests exercise their spiritual gifts, they are connecting with and nurturing one another—each giving and each receiving. Secularists may call this "social discourse," but Christians call this "ministry"—the ministry of being Christ to one another.

Drawing from the neuroscience perspective, social discourse requires multiple brain functions, which, apparently, are dedicated just to the social situations.[21] Zull states:

> One aspect of the brain, learning theory, and knowledge is that it is about the living person. About people. This social element is of great importance in effective learning. *People remember their experience with others more than any other delivery method or isolated searches.*[22]

Zull continues by affirming the role of individual assignments and isolated study, including the use of technology. But he notes that many people prefer their learning through social media because it is more socially interactive thus promoting greater stimulation of the brain. The image of learners hovering over their computers all day has been turned upside down just within this decade. In concluding his book, Zull then says that peoples' "natural social instincts . . . remain important and powerful. I mention this here because it illustrates the potential for more integration of both group work and isolated work. Both are important for the development of the mind."[23]

We have been emphasizing the role of open questions, discussion/dialog, debriefing, rehearsal of content, community learning, and other social dimensions of learning. The priesthood of all believers means that we reach out into the community of believers and unbelievers and engage them with the grace of God with whatever abilities and gifts God has given us. It also means that we exercise our priesthood in our classrooms, Bible study groups and Sunday school classes, youth meetings, mentoring, discipleship, and in the home—especially the home, where every voice, every priest, deserves to be part of the discourse. All of these venues will be superior learning environments if we exercise our priestly function of speaking into one another's lives and inviting others to speak into ours. Please remember, everyone is a priest. There is no hierarchy, only mutuality. We each give and receive without partiality.

I attend a very interactive community women's Bible study in a home. The women who attend come from different churches, some are new believers, and the occasional one doesn't attend church at all. Given the nature of the group, we expect to hear some questions and comments that stray from biblical truth or may even border on heresy. When this happens, I tend to watch for the inevitable gentle response from one of the believers nudging the group back to a biblical perspective. To her great credit, JoAnn, the study leader (a woman with immense biblical knowledge) generally waits to see if someone else in the group will bring us back to a Bible passage or answer the question on the table. Finally, her willingness to be transparent by sharing her own life experience contributes to our sense of safety within the group. Thus, every week, I see the priesthood of all believers operating so beautifully under the guidance of the Holy Spirit.

Summary of Learning Tasks to Begin Practice

1. Once learners have begun to practice their new behaviors it should be followed by a debriefing of their initial attempts. How did it feel? What barriers did they encounter? What helped them to continue practicing?

2. Remind them of the power of the word *yet*. "I may not be getting it right . . . yet."

3. Encourage consistent practice over time since regular repetition strengthens the neural networks that sustain the new behavior.

4. Create a supportive, interactive learning community where people can be honest about their failures and receive encouragement and help in problem solving. In other words, practice the priesthood of all believers.

5. Be honest with the learners about your own successes and failures, and model a supportive attitude. Authenticity and transparency foster safety and freedom.

Encourage learners to search the Scripture for strength to persist and pray for and with each other.

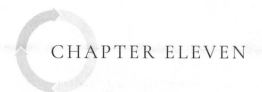

CHAPTER ELEVEN

Learning Tasks
Leading to Practice

My mother and brothers are those who hear God's word and put it into practice.

JESUS, LUKE 8:21

To be is to do.

SOCRATES

Who is wise and understanding among you? Let them show it by their good life,
by deeds done in the humility that comes from wisdom.

JAMES 3:13

THE CRITICAL CHALLENGE in Recall with Practice is making a clear connection between the truth and practice of the truth. Only when the learner grasps the connection between truth and living and begins to practice the truth can we confidently assume that learning has actually occurred.

Both of us have attended Bible school, and Duane also attended seminary. Bible schools and seminaries tend to affirm the application of truth to life and practice. In fact, they are rigorous about requiring students to be engaged in some type of ministry during the entire time in school. One semester in Bible school, both Duane and I were assigned to the same weekly ministry in what is known as "skid row," reaching out to street people. In fact, that is where we first met. Each week we traveled to the ministry venue by train, ministered there, and completed a checklist report on the experience.

As we look back on it, we realize now no one ever asked us to connect what was happening in our ministry to our classes. No one ever asked us about what we were doing in ministry, what we were learning as we practiced ministry, or how it connected to what we were learning in our classes. These two experiences were two parallel railroad tracks that never met. Both faculty and administration sincerely hoped that we were making those connections on our own. Occasionally by God's grace we did. But most of the time, these two—classes and ministry—were completely isolated from each other. It was a faulty assumption. Teachers did not ask about our ministry, and ministry administrators never asked about either our classes or our ministry apart from seeing the report (mostly related to numbers) we handed in to the office each week.

Not until we both attended MSU, a land grant university created to apply science to real world problems, did we fully grasp the impact of teachers helping to make connections between content and life. Earlier, as nursing professor, I had certainly understood the power of a nursing curriculum that expected the students to apply content they were learning to case studies and finally to use that content with actual patients in the hospital. However, not until my graduate work at MSU did I fully understand that *all* education, not just nursing principles, should have this goal in mind. Our learners should not be expected to make all these connections to life without an educator's help.

EDUCATIONAL APPROACHES TO PRACTICE

Since educators are convinced that practice is critical for behavior to change, how can we design and promote practice and connect practice to truth? There are several approaches a teacher can use to incorporate practice into the learning environment.

Social simulations. Using social simulations provides one approach to help learners practice new behaviors. Simulations (sometimes called learning games) set up social situations along with minimal rules for acting in that situation. Social simulations can be employed either before or after certain content has been presented. For example, in our cross-cultural training we often used the "blind walk" to introduce the concept of trust. We would pair people up, have one close his or her eyes and keep them closed while the other led the person around (holding one arm for safety) in silence for a period of minutes. At a certain signal, they would switch roles and the former "blind" person would be the leader for the same amount of time. When we debrief their experience with questions, the students themselves almost never fail to surface most of the trust concepts we had hoped they were experiencing and learning. (A note of caution: I once tried this with a group of junior high students. They got into the simulation so completely that I had put a stop to "leading" the "blind" person under cars and through puddles. However, one lesson in trust they did learn thoroughly was how to go about breaking trust. Then we had to work on rebuilding trust.)

The beauty of using a simulation is that it invariably captures both the cognitive and the affective (feeling) dimension. Consequently, learners are fully engaged in the experience and are quick to share their experiences. The emotional dimension, you will recall, was described earlier in Level II: Recall with Appreciation as the "gateway to learning."

Besides tapping into the learners' affective response, another purpose of a social simulation is to move learners into the application or action phase, where they have the opportunity to observe and then reflect on their own actions and decide the best way to act in real life.

Other simulations illustrated. Earlier you read about a Sunday school class of high school juniors who were confronted with the realities of new marriages. Each group had to write what conditions contributed to their re-spective "marriage" situation. This was an example of a very simple social simulation. Monopoly has also been a popular simulation. Historically a group of high-level business people gathered each year in London, England, to play Monopoly for three days. Observers report that the players played Monopoly similar to the way they conducted their business. Businesses use simulations extensively in corporate training. In fact, the business section of a bookstore usually has the best selection of simulations and gaming books. Perhaps easier, do a search on your computer using those terms.

Because simulations are so powerful in revealing a person's values, they are now being used in research studies to unmask those values. And why are values important? They tend to drive people's behavior.[1]

However, in a learning context it is absolutely key that the learners themselves get to reflect on their own behavior and their values after the simulation ends. Otherwise, they are unlikely to learn anything from the simulated experience.

Open questions about what happened include these: How did you feel about what happened? What have you learned from this exercise? Would you do anything differently next time (speculation)? These prompt learners to examine their own behavior and their values.[2] Failure to ask open questions results in random comments with little learning.

Years ago we used the Ungame to help church people reflect on their lives, build relationships within the group, and connect life experience with God's word. The Ungame is described as "a non-competitive learning/communication board game" that fosters the "serious exchange of thoughts, feelings and ideas."[3] We played it as a board game but emphasized the answers to the questions on the cards. This subtle adjustment stimulated greater thought and discussion. While Duane pastored a church, we used the Ungame questions in a multigenerational group. One middle school boy drew a question about his greatest fear. With hesitancy he told us that the previous day he had been diagnosed with a potentially debilitating disease, the same as his father had struggled with his entire adult life. He was very afraid, and rightfully so. The group reached out to that child with empathy and encouragement, prayed for him, and continued to pray for him long after the game finished. Today he is well into his adult years and the disease is being controlled.

Debriefing simulations. In more complex social simulations in the classroom, learners are allowed to freely make choices and take actions as they see fit given the framework laid out ahead of time. After the simulation is concluded, in the debriefing session learners must be given the chance to reflect on the actions they took, the values undergirding those actions and the consequences of those actions. Only then are they free to consider whether they made the best choices or wish they had acted differently. If not carefully debriefed, a simulation will accomplish nothing.

Debriefing is critical to learning.[4] Good debriefing draws a direct connection between truth and action, content and behavior, the cognitive and the psychomotor. The best learning tends to occur when you think about how you behaved during the simulation, how others behaved, and the consequences. Learners encounter a disorienting dilemma, feelings arise, actions are chosen, and the consequences of those actions are experienced. The debriefing questions allow learners to reflect upon and finally assess whether they were pleased or disappointed (more disorientation) with their behavior. New ideas emerge and the Learning Cycle repeats itself.

Some people tend to dismiss a simulation as "just a game" and deny the power of a simulation to expose their typical behavior. However, habitual behavior patterns are not that easily masked. While the occasional person may "step out of their values," it is not typical. More likely it could be a form of denial—the inability to face their real self.

Although simulations contribute to practicing a new skill, a well-run simulation often creates new disorienting dilemmas, which then trigger a new cycle of transformative learning stages as described by Mezirow. In this sense, the Learning Cycle should be seen as a spiral. For, in the process of beginning to practice and integrate new truths and behaviors into our lives, those very measures sometimes create new disorienting dilemmas that then require reflection on other assumptions and the Learning Cycle begins all over again. See the final chapter for thoughts on how the Learning Cycle can spiral into new learning.

In a well-designed and well-run simulation, the learners freely act out their values in a nonjudgmental social environment and are then, during the debriefing, given the freedom to reflect critically on what they have learned. The beauty of social system simulations is that they allow learners to discover truths for themselves, leading to more acute learning because it includes both practice and emotion, the two elements that will cause neural networks to form and grow in the brain.[5]

Another social simulation that we have used over the years with excellent learning effects has been what is known as the "Broken Squares" simulation.[6]

The purpose of Broken Squares is to help people experience a group problem solving situation. Then in the debriefing, they are asked to analyze their own behaviors: Which did or, did not, contribute to solving the problem? Broken Squares invariably creates considerable reflection and surfaces unconscious assumptions and surprising perspectives as people share their thoughts and experience in the debriefing. It is also very helpful when played with cross-cultural groups because different cultures tend to approach problems

> *Educational games have the potential to help students reach important educational goals such as acquiring important foundational knowledge.*
>
> CLAIRE HOWELL MAJOR, MICHAEL S. HARRIS, AND TODD ZAKRAJSEK, *TEACHING FOR LEARNING*

differently. Just a note of caution when using any social system simulation: always test the simulation first on a group of friends in order to give yourself some idea how it works and what will be the learning payoff.

We have found simulations to be very useful in stimulating interest in a topic and in helping people "see themselves." Sometimes reality itself forces us to see ourselves and initiate appropriate change. A group of people in a training program once decided to play volleyball to have fun and relax. A range of people from elderly to middle school participated. One young man joined and turned out to be skillful and competitive. As the ball came to his side of the net, he would rush into someone's space to hit the ball back, bumping people and knocking children aside. This went on for maybe fifteen minutes. One could see the disorienting dilemma. But what to do?

At one point the athlete hit the ball over the net and a tall fellow who could easily have reached out and hit it back said, "Hey, Johnny, get it." Johnny, about eleven years old, took a powerful swing and hit the ball off to the side causing a loss of a point. The tall fellow, who could have easily hit it back, stepped over to Johnny, gently patted him on the head, and said, "That was a great try." Then this same tall man ran off to the side, picked up the ball and, as he tossed it back to the other side, said, "I'd rather lose a point than a child." *What brilliance*, I thought. From that point, the game changed. Everyone played cooperatively and all had fun. That innocent game contained a lifelong lesson.

Skills training with built-in practice. In addition to simulations, a second educational approach to practice is what we call skills training with built-in practice. During my years teaching in the educational studies PhD program at Trinity International University, a recurring theme in classes was the skill of facilitating discussion, a necessary skill for any educator, mentor, or Bible study leader who teaches using interactive methods.

Interactive teaching invariably engages the learners and generates discussion. Any teacher wishing to inspire students toward competent practice must sprinkle probing open questions throughout her or his class notes. Questions stimulate reflection and discussion and, especially, draw students "back in" to a lecture that may have gone beyond the fifteen to seventeen minutes for prime-time attention. (See chapter three for Sousa's retention chart.)

Student responses to open questions very often expose misunderstandings, misinformation, or even outright falsehoods that they hold. Those responses also allow the students to express their understanding of a concept in their own words, thus retrieving content and strengthening neural connections. In essence, open questions are learning tasks to provoke the learners to think, to capture and hold their attention, and to relate the content to their own life situation.

Creating open questions that stimulate discussion of content is just the easy part. Facilitating all the responses to those questions, making sure discussion stays productive (and out of the weeds), assuring participants equal voice, helping people build on each other's ideas, avoiding meaningless monologues, maintaining a safe environment for the timid—all the while encouraging authentic dialogue—is like grasping the proverbial tiger by the tail. Facilitating discussion is a complex skill. The challenges are enormous and that is precisely why so many professors are intimidated at the thought of trying to facilitate a productive discussion in the classroom. They fear what they have seen too often: a session where people simply share off topic, meaninglessly and superficially.

I started every PhD course by creating, together with the student input, a list of guidelines for discussion, which I posted at the front of the class every class period. We listed such items as these: build on each other's ideas; be constructive in your feedback; do not interrupt; be brief in your comments, and so on. Still students would say to me, "You make it look so easy, but when I try it in my teaching, I find it so difficult." It may be difficult to facilitate good discussion, but you will get better and the rewards are enormous. There is no substitute for getting students to think, to reason, to speculate, and then to begin the change their lives.

Obviously, facilitating discussion takes practice—and a good deal of practice at that. How does an educator go about learning and teaching such a complex skill? Yet if you think about it, facilitating discussion is so critical for leading people to the truth. I have seen it done. Read on.

Skills training with built-in practice illustrated. A couple of years ago, I saw this built-in-practice training approach to facilitating discussion work exquisitely. The organization Entrust invited me to sit in on one of their training modules as a consultant.[7] Entrust has a profound kingdom impact on churches in the United States and globally. Churches that send small groups of volunteer men and women to Entrust workshops for training see these individuals become a force for the gospel as they begin using their ministry skills within the church and community.

The particular training module they asked me to observe was called "Facilitating Relational Learning" (FRL). A module description states that it "explores the unique needs of the adult learner and how facilitating discussions in a relational context can be a powerful way to not only introduce content but stimulate growth that leads to mature disciples of Jesus Christ."[8]

A small group of only six women (Entrust also offers this training for men) spent five days together learning how to facilitate Bible studies. Previous experience in group facilitation was not required. The only requirement was a reading assignment and a willingness to learn. By the end of our time together, each of those six women had almost flawlessly facilitated a full forty-minute Bible study for the rest of us.

How did our two Entrust teachers accomplish that? Here's what I observed:

- Our two teachers never failed to model highly interactive facilitation skills.

- All content centered on Jesus' teaching methods, best practices in the field of adult education, and the exploration of many rich Scripture passages.

- We were taught how to ask the group what they expected from their time together; how to give everyone equal opportunity to speak; and how to explore the relevance of the topic to daily life.

Early on, each learner began conducting her assigned practice session (between twenty and forty minutes) with the rest of us acting as the Bible study group. Each was assigned a different topic of spiritual growth with a focus on the Scripture for her session. Timing devices were used to time each session. After each practice session, together we all evaluated the session, following certain rules to ensure that our comments were both safe and constructive.

By the end of the five days, each woman had conducted three full practice sessions, which were immediately evaluated by herself and the group. Three practice sessions for each of six women meant that altogether the group witnessed eighteen full practice sessions and evaluations.

The genius of the curricular design was the gradual introduction of only one or two critical facilitation skills for each practice session. For example, Sherry Bohn, one of our two Entrust teachers, describes the second practice session this way:

> The facilitator is only allowed to ask questions. This forces the leader to listen, to think more deeply about powerful open questions to guide the discussion,

and to realize that the Holy Spirit can teach the group key concepts without hearing a lecture about the facilitator's 'nugget.'[9]

Each woman was amazed at how well her group session had gone even though all she could do was to ask open questions. She was not permitted to make even one of her own comments! Having once learned the disciplines of asking, listening, thinking, and further asking, later they were permitted to add their own thoughts. This question-posing discipline addressed one of the big difficulties in building facilitations skills, the leader's "need" to share all they know—along with the usual anxiety that builds with the silence that ensues when members are thinking about how to respond to the question.

On the last day together, for the final practice assignments, each woman showed that she was completely comfortable and competent as she facilitated the Bible study.

A great deal more could be written about the way in which our Entrust teachers helped their learners grow into skilled facilitators. We included their approach as an excellent example of how to build ministry skills.

The participants found the learning environment to be safe, relational, interactive, and content-focused (the content being mainly Scripture). These women also learned the power of and the skill of posing open questions, respecting time limits, making studies relevant to their learners, and a host of other skills taught and modeled throughout the week. Most impressive was that each woman left that week having competently demonstrated a superb capability to facilitate a

> *Failure(s) . . . too often characterized as a negative . . . , (are) opportunities in disguise, valuable gifts misidentified as tragedy.*
>
> JESSICA LAHEY, *THE GIFT OF FAILURE*

Bible study. If you are curious, I recommend you explore further all of Entrust's excellent opportunities for ministry training.[10]

The gift of failure. What if the first few attempts at new behavior are colossal failures? What to do then? In no way does this affirm a shoddy approach to practice. It requires a careful assessment of what went wrong and the attempt to do it better next time.

The chapter on barriers suggested that one strategy for successful behavior change was to identify potential barriers before attempting to practice the behavior. A second strategy for success was also noted. When early attempts to perform the new behavior fail, and often they do, how should we proceed? A strategic time to analyze what might have caused us to fail is immediately after the failure. Failure can be a reason to give up, or it can become a powerful learning tool on the way to achieving success.

In the Entrust illustration above, note that every practice session, all eighteen of them, was followed by an evaluation—both a self and a peer evaluation. More often evaluation is known by a less intimidating term—*feedback*. Feedback offers a new opportunity to hone a particular skill. Good feedback must contain the provision that it is both safe and constructive. Entrust ensured that the evaluation or feedback times were safe by asking the facilitator herself to be the first to express what she had done well and what needed improvement. Safety also required that feedback given by peers and the facilitator was constructive. And so, their facilitation skills were honed during each session. Not only did the practicing facilitator learn from the feedback session herself, but every one of her group members learned how to improve during each practice session.

But what about the time expenditure? Many will argue that this model of skills training takes way too much time, energy, and expense. And, because it *does* require all of that, teachers will often settle for less. They will do their best to list the facilitation skills, discuss them in depth, and model good facilitation practices before their learners. Then they hope their learners will somehow be persistent enough to actually practice the skills in their own classrooms. From my experience, rarely does this happen. If you believe a skill is important and needs to be developed, then it is worth the time and expense to make sure the learner can perform it competently. The question remains: How critical is the skill or the behavior you hope the learner will integrate into life? If critical, then what amount of practice and follow-up is worth it to build that behavior into their own lives?

Alternating practice with regular debriefing. Along with social simulations and skills training with built-in practice, a third educational approach that encourages practice and develops competency is alternating practice with regular debriefing. This approach is often seen in regular weekly church Bible study groups, small groups, and discipleship groups.

Unfortunately, most weekly church group leaders simply teach Biblical truths and may even suggest implications for daily practice, but rarely do they actively encourage people to decide to change their behavior. A simple presentation of a Biblical truth by the leader without further exploration and discussion of the practical implications too often falls on busy, distracted ears (the seed falling among the thorns). It is a rare person who, once at home, does the hard work of reflecting on truth heard in the group, thinks about how to incorporate that truth into life, and then decides to try and take action. In the next chapter on Recall with Habit, we describe a Sunday school teacher who chose to follow this approach.

A group leader who hopes to promote transformative learning will pose provocative open questions. These questions can nudge the learners to think about how a truth could impact their own life, then ask what steps they could take in the next week to build that truth into their daily activity. Such group reflection presupposes transparent, safe, and free flowing conversations. Here the group leader must bear the full responsibility for creating safety and transparency.

In the next group meeting the leader would be wise to debrief those who attempted to make any changes during the previous week. Neglecting to specifically debrief any changes a person tried to make during the previous week is a huge missed opportunity to consolidate learning, celebrate what went well, and talk about failure as a "lesson learned."

> *Results! Why, man, I have gotten a lot of results! I know several thousand things that won't work.*
>
> THOMAS EDISON

Another illustration of alternating practice with debriefing follows. Several years ago, GATE (Global Associates for Transformational Education) was formed by four of us who had training and experience both as faculty and administration. Most important, we (Duane) shared a common educational philosophy, the kind you are reading about in this book. Our three-day workshops used an abundance of open questions such as: "Describe the students coming to your school (training program)." "What do you want your graduates to look like when they leave?" "Describe the church ministry context they will be entering."

Their answers to the questions provided the early *content* (recall from their observations). Their answers generated relevance, value, and expectation (*affect*) that easily fed into *speculation*. "How does your teaching (classes) contribute to preparing them, given who they are when they come and who you would like them to be when they leave?" "Is there more that can be done? If so, what?" "What difficulties might you confront if you followed through (practice) on your thoughts about 'What can I do?'"

As workshop leaders we had to struggle with the sustainability concern: *recall with habit*. We had everyone write their plan for a change they believed would help them do better in their educational goals. They shared them with each other and wrote their ideas on poster paper that was taped on the wall for everyone to see. Then we told them that the following year we would ask them what they had done, and how it had worked. A year later we debriefed them on the changes made. (Note: Each level of the Learning Cycle was involved in this workshop.)

Role play. Role play is a fourth approach to build practice into a learning event along with simulations, skills training with built in practice, and alternating practice with regular debriefing. We introduced role play in the barriers chapter as a way to help learners deal with a barrier that could keep them from doing what they know is the right thing to do. So we mention it briefly here because it can also provide an opportunity for practice as well, under the guidance of the teacher. When set up properly, role play can help the learner begin to feel what it is like to take those first action steps toward change and to practice the new behavior.

LEARNING TASKS RESPECT HOW THE BRAIN LEARNS

Each of the above educational approaches is designed to strengthen practice but also to respect how the brain learns. Each approach adheres to the following learning principles that strengthen and grow neural networks in the brain.

Safety. The rational, or reasoning, part of the brain functions best when the learner's emotional state is one of feeling valued, being safe, being respected. A mind relatively free of fear of embarrassment, of criticism, of being misunderstood can fully engage the content and consider its meaning for life.

Repetition. The brain values repetition because the information stored is available for immediate use, meaning the brain functions become more efficient. The same is true for behavior that becomes habitual. Habit is nothing more than repetition of a behavior until it becomes "automatic," which is not to say "robotic."

Rehearsal. Every time a learner returns to a thought, considers it more carefully, and gains an insight, neural networks are stimulated to grow and become stronger. In addition to the rehearsal activities noted earlier, debriefing of individual behavior within a social simulation or after a week of practice is one of the more powerful forms of rehearsal. It encourages learners to evaluate their own behavior in light of the content being presented.

Engagement. Absolutely nothing happens in the brain if the learner is not engaged or thinking about the topic. The provision of a dialogical community (like a Bible study group or a skill training event) where problems can be solved and actions revisited and evaluated promotes engagement at the highest level.[11]

Action. With every action, changes occur in the brain. Neural networks broaden, strengthen, and initiate more connecting pathways. Each action taken makes it easier to repeat the behavior next time and to form a habit.

One woman who was part of our Facilitating Relational Learning group at Entrust was a missionary in Papua New Guinea. She returned to the mission field and reported to the rest of us how she was using her new facilitation skills for teaching Bible to the women in the village.

SUMMARY OF LEARNING TASKS

So, what are teachers to do in order to help learners navigate Level IV: Recall with Practice?

1. Design an educational setting where people expect to be challenged and debriefed on their actual attempts to put God's truths into practice.

2. Be intentional about calling people to explore what changes God is calling them to make in their lives; encourage them to decide to do something about it now and then follow up on how that trial went.

3. Encourage realistic goals with small incremental steps for each goal to help learners avoid failure. For example, say someone decides to practice regular reading of the Scripture and prayer. They may decide to do this daily between 4:00 and 6:00 am. If they have not practiced this spiritual discipline before, and especially if they are not "morning people," they

are going to find this goal quite a challenge. And if they fail, they will be unlikely to try again. Most tend to say, "Been there. Done that. Doesn't work!" It is best to start with small goals—challenging but not that difficult—and then with success, set higher goals later on.

4. Be prepared with open questions to explore feelings (possibly negative) related to how early practices played out. And then follow-up first with affirmation for the courage it took to attempt the change. Then continue with questions about what could have gone better and how to improve. Not everyone is good at creating probing, open questions in the moment. I have learned to prepare them before I need them. Then I can relax and watch the learners get engaged in the challenge.

5. Listen carefully for real and potential barriers and discuss ways to overcome them.

6. Allow time for problem solving related to barriers they are encountering in their practice.

7. Where appropriate, encourage learners to build accountability relationships.

Once practice becomes a habit, it becomes much easier to sustain as a new behavior. And then it becomes a part of your identity. The habit becomes integral to who you are . . . to God's glory. Responsible practice is rooted in recall, motivated by affect, formed by speculation, and forged by analyzing the barriers.

This next chapter explores how habits are formed and become integral to a person's life and character.

Recall with Habit

I do consistently

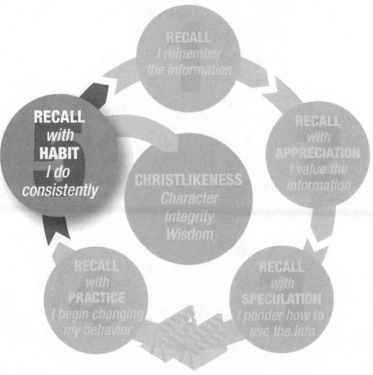

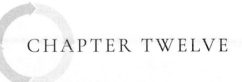

CHAPTER TWELVE

Building a Habit

Do not conform to the pattern of this world, but be transformed by the renewing of your mind. Then you will be able to test and approve what God's will is—his good, pleasing and perfect will.

ROMANS 12:2

Education isn't teaching people to know what they don't know. It is teaching them to behave as they don't behave.

UNKNOWN

To hold to a doctrine or an opinion with the intellect alone is not to believe it. A man's real belief is that which he lives by.

GEORGE MACDONALD, *KNOWING THE HEART OF GOD*

K NOWLEDGE HAS IMPLICATIONS for how we conduct our lives. Becoming a more competent, integrated, and mature human being calls for acting in light of new learning until our lives are transformed in specific areas. A transformed life presupposes new thinking, new attitudes, and new behaviors so automatic and so instinctual that they now characterize the person we have become. And so, we come to Level V: Recall with Habit.

SHEEP AND GOATS

In Jesus' parable of the sheep and the goats, neither group had any idea that when they encountered a person who was "hungry . . . thirsty . . . stranger . . . naked . . . sick . . . or in prison" that they were meeting Christ himself (Mt 25: 35-36 NKJV). But the sheep showed compassion and the goats withheld it. Why? In Skye Jethani's words, the sheep were living "integrated" lives.

> The righteous do not segment their lives into categories of "sacred" and "ordinary;" they do not view some activities or people as important to God and others as unimportant. . . . Their love for God flows into all aspects of their lives including how they see and act toward the least. Justice marks all of their relationships.

The goats, on the other hand, were living "dis-integrated" lives because "their commitment to Christ was dis-integrated from other parts of their existence."[1]

The Pharisees and teachers of the law (Level II: Recall) lived dis-integrated lives—thus, Jesus' charge of hypocrisy. They were not who they claimed to be. Their words sounded right, but in their being they were corrupt "goats" leading dis-integrated lives—fractured lives, isolating truth from the flow of life.

Daily we are all being transformed to some degree. Each new truth we learn and consider valuable must be weighed for consequences—good or bad—along with the difficulty of putting it into practice. We must be convinced that the end result will be rewarding or we won't even try to change. Change requires doing something consistently over time for a new habit to be formed. It takes determination and discipline to incorporate these new thoughts, attitudes, and actions. Only after some time do we realize they have come to fit comfortably into our lifestyle. This final goal of good learning we have called Level V: Recall with Habit—"I do consistently." Integrity grows with consistency. What we know is being integrated into our daily thoughts and actions. Habits become who we are. Character is being formed. The person who sees God's truth and obeys is defined in Scripture as a "wise" person (Mt 7:24).[2] The Greek word (*phronimos*) Mathew uses for "wise" has the thrust of prudent and discerning use of knowledge.

God's truth has consequences. It demands that not only do we acknowledge it (recall, rehearse, remember) but that we order our lives in accordance with it. Doing something consistently over time results in a habit. Resist letting the awkward feelings discourage you as you practice a new habit. Certainly do not quit. If it is the right thing to do, then persevere. Over time that new habit will feel comfortable, normal, and right. It is starting to be integral to who we are and who we are becoming.

WHAT IS A HABIT?

Researchers have identified the components of a habit and the process by which habits are created or changed. McKeown cites Duke University researchers who found that "40% of the choices we make each day are deeply unconscious."[3] These daily routines repeat so often, and the neural networks are now so developed that our brain simply automates them. This automation requires much less effort. For example, think about our habit of walking. For most of us it is automatic. But what if you had to tell one leg to move forward and then tell the other to do the same, and then do it all over again? Think of the energy required. The brain strives for efficiency so it can concentrate on more difficult tasks. Habits allow the brain to go on "cruise control."

> *We must literally change the criteria for (educational) success. Our goal should be a spontaneous demonstration of habits of the mind.*
>
> JAMES E. ZULL, *FROM BRAIN TO MIND*

A habit then, is a specific recurring thought behavior or set of behaviors that have become so automatic that we can repeat them without thinking. A habit is a default setting. It becomes an integral part of who we are. Our brains instinctually draw on these "effort-saving" routines in order to focus elsewhere, says Duhigg in *The Power of Habit: Why We Do What We Do in Life and Business.*[4]

For example, we worked hard to teach our two sons, while still toddlers, to look a person in the eye whenever they were spoken to or whenever they spoke to someone. Meeting the eyes of another person in conversation demonstrates both attention and respect within our Western culture. It draws people to you and invites engagement. If you have ever parented a child, you know it requires considerable persistence—many reminders—and enormous encouragement until such a routine is established. Now, many years later, I smile inside as I watch these two men habitually look directly at anyone who engages them in conversation.

HOW ARE HABITS FORMED?

Duhigg summarizes what we currently know about habit formation. A habit consists of three things: (1) the *cue*, a trigger or hint "that tells your brain to go into automatic mode and which habit to use," (2) the *routine*, or set of behaviors that constitute the habit, which can be physical, mental, or emotional, and (3) the *reward*, which often consists of a "sense of accomplishment" triggering the release of "endorphins" such as dopamine and serotonin into our blood stream. Endorphins produce positive emotions, sometimes even a "high." Positive emotions stimulate an interest in and desire to repeat the experience. For example, being acknowledged for "a job well done" sparks a motivation to keep on doing well. This would be an intrinsic reward, the kind that usually promotes long-term behavior. "Extrinsic rewards, money, prizes, stars, badges may be used to encourage the start of new habits but usually work best in the short term."[5]

Many studies demonstrate that for a habit to endure, a person must eventually begin to "expect" and then "crave" the reward.[6] In fact, once a habit is well established, a dopamine spike tends to occur at the cue reinforcing the habit even before the routine behavior starts. Thus, we begin to crave the habit routine as soon as the cue appears. In fact, neuroscientists such as Sapolsky, have discovered that once well-established, a cue can cause the brain to begin to release more dopamine in anticipation of the reward than is released by the reward itself.[7]

Habits are feedback loops that we run over and over until a behavior occurs without conscious thought.

DAVID DiSALVO, *BRAIN CHANGER*

Duhigg explains further:

> Researchers have learned that cues can be almost anything, from a visual trigger such as a candy bar or a television commercial to a certain place, a time of day, an emotion, a sequence of thoughts, or the company of particular people. Routines can be incredibly complex or fantastically simple. . . . Rewards can range from food or drugs that cause physical sensations, to emotional payoffs, such as the feelings of pride that accompany praise or self-congratulation.[8]

For example, Duane's physician told him to work on his posture in order to prevent getting "humped over." So, each night after brushing his teeth, he stands straight against the wall for two minutes. It seems to be working. Brushing his teeth is the cue that "standing against the wall is next." The reward is better posture and feeling good about what he is accomplishing. This process of connecting one habit to another, or "habit stacking," will ensure the new habit will stick.[9]

As we deliberately and consistently choose to act in certain ways in response to specific situations, our brains gradually begin to automate that behavior loop and a habit is born. Such daily habits smooth out our lives by literally linking hundreds of automatic routines to free us to deal with more important issues. Habits help us do what we need to do quickly without much thought. So we drive, eat, brush our teeth, play video games, and check email all without much (if any) forethought and planning. The cue, routine, and reward all merge into daily living habits that streamline our lives. We hear the phone text ding, glance at the message, and feel a connection with the person who sent the text. Because they have become automatic, habits often roll out in our behavior unconsciously—outside of our awareness.

Duhigg also reminds us that habits can form "without our permission."[10] Somewhere in our past we made unthinking choices and took actions that become habit routines. Then one day, some event (perhaps a class you attended or the reminder of a friend) raised the hidden habit to our awareness and we suddenly recognized, there it was—a fully formed habit! Then, once recognized, we can decide whether it helps or harms and what to do about it. Habits can form anywhere at any time, with effort or sometimes without our knowledge.

These unconscious habits can themselves create surprising barriers to the change we intend to make. It isn't until we decide to change, step out into a new way of thinking or acting, and then fall flat on our face that we begin to suspect that something beyond our consciousness is happening.

> *If we create a routine that enshrines the essentials, we will begin to execute them on autopilot . . . it will happen without our having to think about it.*
>
> GREG McKEOWN, *ESSENTIALISM*

That even requires careful reflection and sometimes even the helpful observations of a teacher, a classmate, or a good friend to raise those invisible habits to
our awareness. Speculating ahead of time which barriers could arise can often
help us avoid failure later as discussed in Level III: Recall with Speculation—"I
ponder how to use the information." But sometimes it takes a few attempts to
act and fail before the barriers become clear. Here is where supportive teachers,
classmates, and learning groups who ask penetrating questions are absolutely
critical to achieving and sustaining valuable life changes.

HABITS ARE PART OF BEING HUMAN

In his biography of Christian leader John Stott, Roger Steer reminds us that

> what we are is partly the result of creation (the image of God) and partly the
> result of the fall (the image defaced). The self we are to deny, disown and
> crucify is our fallen self, everything within us that is incompatible with Jesus
> Christ. The self we are to affirm and value is our created self, everything within
> us that is compatible with Jesus Christ. True self-denial (the denial of our false,
> fallen self) is not the road to self-destruction but the road to self-discovery.[11]

When God created us human beings, he equipped us with this marvelous
predisposition to form habits. The Bible affirms that we are created in the
image of God (Gen 1:26, 27). Our tendency to form habits is part of how we
were created and how we operate as human beings. Unfortunately, the Bible
also affirms humankind's fall into sin, where that magnificent image of God
was defaced and distorted within each of us. The Eastern Orthodox church
uses the metaphor of a "mirror" to represent the image of God. Like a mirror,
the image of God reflects the beauty of Christ himself to the world. Sin
"shatters" that mirror and covers it with "cracks and fissures," making it hard
to see Christ himself.[12]

Consequently, the fall introduced negative habit formation. But re-
demption through Christ opened the way for godly habit formation and restoration of the image of God.

Jesus Christ knew the power of good life habits and faithfully included
them into his daily life. The gospel stories record them. Both Mark and Luke
tell us he often withdrew to pray early in the morning and preferred to pray
in lonely places and on mountainsides (Mk 1:35; Lk 5:16). They tell us that he
usually attended a synagogue on the Sabbath and often taught there (Mk 1:21;

Lk 4:16; 13:10). Jesus routinely healed people, responded to their questions, and taught about the kingdom of God. His conduct revealed his character and his values, giving us an ideal picture of what our relationship can be with God our Father. In Jesus' incarnation we catch a glimpse of the perfect human being whose habits were all good and who never gave in to even one sinful habit in spite of the fact that he was tempted like us (Heb 4:15).

> *And what about our bodies that always seemed to come off so badly in every contest with our soul? Did Jesus put on our flesh so that we might despise it?*
>
> WENDELL BERRY, *JAYBER CROW*

GOOD AND BAD HABITS

A good habit moves us forward, builds our confidence, and strengthens our character. Truths we learn can be deliberately integrated into who we are. With God's help we become known for living truthful lives.

Good habit: attitude of gratitude. Recently we attended the memorial of a missionary nurse who gave her life serving the Shona people in Zimbabwe. One colleague called her the "Mother Teresa of Zimbabwe." At the memorial, a niece said her beloved aunt invariably thanked everyone who ever showed her any kindness. The niece said, "My aunt Lorraine had a habit of gratitude." This gracious woman embodied the scriptural injunction "Give thanks in all circumstances; for this is God's will for you in Christ Jesus" (1 Thess 5:18).

Bad habits: poor interpersonal skills and bad attitudes. A bad habit can limit our development, close down our relationships, and weaken our character. Bad habits, as simple as poor interpersonal skills habits, can isolate and discourage us. Or habitual negative attitudes can spiral us down into depressive states that rob us of the joy of living. And we all have encountered people whose lives are virtually destroyed by addictions—bad habits that choke out anything resembling a normal life.

Our brains do not distinguish between good or bad habits. But we do have the capacity to examine our actions and recognize their positive or negative effect on our lives. Bad habits—like snapping in irritation at our spouse, watching too much TV, or eating a large bowl of ice cream every night—can exert just as much power over us as good habits such as getting up every morning to go on a walk. We all have parts of our lives where we fail miserably to do what we know is right and good. James warns all of us, "If anyone, then, knows the good they ought to do and doesn't do it, it is sin for them" (Jas 4:17). Some of us have seriously bad habits that are destroying our relationships with others and God, our capacity to work, and even destroying our very bodies. Replacing sinful habits with godly ones can redeem our lives in spite of painful consequences of the past bad habits.

> *Teachers who use most of their class time lecturing are hoping this style of learning sticks— but it rarely does. Students retain little of what is said.*
>
> ERIC JENSEN, *TEACHING WITH THE BRAIN IN MIND*

Kintsugi. The Japanese art of repairing broken pottery, called *Kintsugi*, offers a lovely picture of what God's redeeming work can look like in our broken lives. In Kintsugi, the artist uses liquid gold to repair a shattered pot. The cracks are still very apparent, but now the pot is whole again and the golden cracks add a peculiar but lovely beauty to the piece itself.

2 Corinthians 4:6-7 states:

> For God, who said, "Let light shine out of darkness," made his light shine in our hearts to give us the light of the knowledge of God's glory displayed in the face of Christ. But we have this treasure in jars of clay to show that this all-surpassing power is from God and not from us.

We are simple clay pots holding this precious light of "the knowledge of God's glory displayed in the face of Christ." And I picture cracks in our pots, our sinful habits, our brokenness, now appear as golden seams where God has healed our broken places with His grace.

Teachers can foster bad habits too. Zull describes how our lectures can "habituate." He writes,

> Nothing demonstrates habituation more than a lecture. Unless we break up the sound every few minutes, we are almost certain to induce habituation in a learner's brain. Even when we think we are breaking it up, we all have "our way" of speaking, and the learner gets used to our way, whatever it is, with time. You may have noticed how interest picks up when a new person begins to talk in a

class or lecture. That interest holds up for a short while, even if the speaker ultimately turns out to be "boring." At first, it is enough that he is new.[13]

Earlier in chapter four we discussed the importance of creating lectures that hold learners' attention. We cannot overemphasize the importance of creating changeups (breaks—at least every fifteen to seventeen minutes) in our lectures so as to keep the learners interested and engaged. So many truths evaporate into oblivion once learners become habituated to the sound of a lecturer's voice.

How to Replace a Bad Habit

Researchers remind us we can be intentional about replacing a bad habit with a good habit. By thinking carefully about new truths we hope to incorporate into our daily lives, we can build on our tendency to form habits. A teacher's goal, then, is to guide the learners to align their thinking, emotions, attitudes, and actions with new information that can transform their lives.

Be encouraged. Our brains can be rewired. People learn new ways of being and acting all the time. Sometimes new habits need to be formed and other times an old habit needs to be replaced or revised. When a habit needs to be revised, the same cue and reward should be kept while the routine (the behavior) is replaced.

> *Once you understand that habits can change, you have the freedom—and the responsibility—to remake them.*
>
> CHARLES DUHIGG, *THE POWER OF HABIT*

Life Lesson Learned

Several years ago, our pastor asked me (Muriel) to present our Learning Cycle to the church adult Bible teachers who were starting a new term of Sunday school classes. In that group was a biology professor from our local Christian college. Challenged by the Learning Cycle model, he announced that he was going to teach an adult Sunday school class on Matthew 6 using the model. I was intrigued and signed up for the class.

Dr. Fred Van Dyke titled his first Sunday school class "An Audience of One" because Jesus in Matthew 6 tells his followers not to "practice your righteousness in front of others to be seen by them" (Mt 6:1) but to do it "in secret.

Then your Father, who sees what is done in secret, will reward you" (Mt 6:4). The righteous deeds to be done in secret were giving to the needy, praying to the Father (which includes the Lord's prayer), fasting, storing up treasures in heaven, and not being anxious.

During the first class, Fred told us what to expect. He would spend one class discussing the first command (giving to the needy). All during the coming week we were to focus on giving to the needy in secret. We were to practice it as best we could, memorize the relevant verses, and come the following week prepared to share what happened. He warned us that he did not plan to teach any new material. The entire class time would focus on our experience over the last week giving to the needy in secret—what we learned and how the week had gone. The irony was not lost on any of us that we were "sharing" what we had done in "secret," but we realized it was an important part of the learning experience. The following week he would discuss the second command (prayer), and on the following Sunday we would share what we learned about praying in secret. The same pattern continued through all of Matthew 6.

As enthusiastic participants, we took the challenge. Each week we practiced the command in question and came ready the following Sunday to share what we had learned from our experience.

When we came to the Lord's Prayer, as usual, I paid special attention to what Jesus said and then I prayed in secret. Around the middle of the week I was stunned to realize that although I had said the Lord's prayer all my life and knew the verses that followed, I was still nursing grudges that went back many years against people who had hurt me. The Scripture was clear: "Forgive us our debts, as we also have forgiven our debtors" (Mt 6:12) and "For if you forgive other people when they sin against you, your heavenly Father will also forgive you. But if you do not forgive others their sins, your Father will not forgive your sins" (Mt 6:14-15).

I asked God to examine my thoughts and point out to me all the people against whom I still held a grudge. He graciously laid out a list for me. One by one, I confessed my sin and determined before God to forgive each person for what they had done. I then asked God to remind me of what I had done whenever I picked up that resentment, that grudge, and began to nurse it all over again. As a person would come to mind, I would remind myself that I had already forgiven that person, reject bitterness and let it go once more.

That was fifteen years ago. Many times, as someone's name popped into my head, I was still tempted to dwell in the pain instead of receiving God's provision of freedom if I freely forgave my debtors. I would have to go before God and reaffirm that I had already forgiven that person. For several months and even years, I found myself repeating the process over and over again. In recent years the resentment towards certain others has had much less of a hold over me. God in His grace has weakened those neural networks.[14]

My disciplined refusal to allow resentment to linger in my thinking (brain) caused that neural network to weaken and the attitude to no longer have that power over me. When neural networks are not stimulated, brain cells die and weaken the network eventually to the point of dysfunction. Those habits we practice generate new brain cells, grow the neural network and become established patterns, even automated patterns. These habits are called "rich experiences" in the literature.[15] For me, this is another example of God's grace as he has made it possible for us to live in peace. It has been a blessed freedom.

I'm still tempted to form new grudges as hurts come my way. But the tendency to soak in them has lessened considerably. A few years ago, Duane led a forgiveness and reconciliation conference in Liberia, West Africa, at the close it its civil war. While considering the atrocities, one Liberian declared, "We must forgive and forget." After a brief pause, another Liberian spoke. "I can forgive but I cannot forget." Another pause occurred before a proverb came forth from yet another voice: "You cannot keep the birds from flying over your head, but you can keep them from building a nest in your hair." A "delete" button in our heads would be nice; but God wants us to remember his forgiveness of our sins and, in remembering, to do the same toward others. The memories will return, true, but we do not need to give them free rent in our heads.

If you consider my experience with forgiveness, it is relatively easy to identify the cue, the routine, and the reward. As a Christian, I developed the habit of confessing my sins and asking God for his forgiveness. This pattern has been part of my daily life since I was in college. The cue or trigger for this habit, as Duhigg terms it, was a recurring sense that I fell short of God's standards in my life and needed to confess my daily sins and receive his forgiveness. The routine, or set of behaviors, was the act of praying, confessing the sins that come to mind, and asking God to forgive me. I then thanked him for his promise of forgiveness. More recent reflection on the Lord's Prayer during the class revealed that I needed to adjust my routine and add forgiving others to this routine. And finally, the reward was the belief that God had indeed forgiven me as he promised, knowing that it pleased him and the hope to become more like Jesus. What further interested me while writing this chapter is the new knowledge from the habit researchers that the reward also includes a release of endorphins into my system. How good is that?

> *Routine is one of the most powerful tools for removing obstacles. Without routine, the pull of nonessential distractions will overpower us.*
>
> GREG McKEOWN, *ESSENTIALISM*

Barriers encountered. What barriers did I encounter when it came to this truth about forgiveness? Here are a couple. In my early days as a Christian, the teaching emphasis had always been about the wonder that God would forgive me if I confessed. But to *be forgiven* also demanded that I also *be a forgiver*, an equal truth rarely taught. I don't remember ever discussing it in depth alongside my being forgiven. But then I encountered a teacher who taught the whole Biblical text in light of our relevant experience. His focus on *my* behavior helped me both recognize and overcome that barrier.

A second barrier was the shame I felt since I had grasped this truth so late in my Christian life. The shame could easily have driven me to minimize the importance of this "aha" moment. I could have shrunk from sharing my experience with the class. Ashamed, I might have persuaded myself that I had always "known" this truth. But in this class, Dr. Van Dyke created a safe environment for us to share our thoughts without judgment. So, I could honestly and authentically share what I had discovered and work through the shame.

Learning Cycle revisited. Let's look at how this fits the Learning Cycle. The Matthew 6 passage on prayer was familiar. I could recall Jesus' truth about forgiveness, even quote the words. But it wasn't enough to change my behavior (Level I: Recall—"I remember the information").

Not until I sat under a Bible teacher who helped me think specifically about the truth as it related to my own life was I able to fully appreciate and value what I was learning. His presentation explored forgiveness in Matthew 6, and the questions he posed for discussion specifically helped us to wrestle with forgiving others as God has forgiven us. Consequently, the full truth about forgiveness suddenly became very relevant to me (Level II: Recall with Appreciation—"I value the information"). Next, we were encouraged to think about how to put the truth into practice as we dialogued about it in class (Level III: Recall with Speculation—"I ponder how to use the information").

Then we spent a week practicing the truth at home (Level IV: Recall with Practice—"I begin changing my behavior"). We returned the following Sunday to talk together about our practice at home and what we had learned. The sharing time accomplished three things for us. First, it caused us to rehearse what we had learned in our attempts to *do* the truth. These were fresh thoughts now as we reported on what we had observed while praying in secret each day. For me, I found myself deliberately attempting to practice forgiveness each day. Remember, rehearsal reactivates and strengthens our brain's neural networks, further ensuring deeper, more sustainable learning. Second, we shared within our learning community the problems (barriers or obstacles) we encountered in our attempts to practice the truth, and we listened to solutions for coping with those problems from each other. And third, our discussion together in the group sharpened our resolve to continue acting on what we had learned.

Before moving on to the next verses in Matthew 6, our Sunday school class had actually spent fourteen days intently focusing on one truth, all the while working hard to incorporate it into our daily experience. Perhaps you have heard that it takes twenty-one days to create a habit. This number was first suggested by Maxwell Maltz in his book *Psycho-Cybernetics* in 1960. The scientific data since then suggests a more realistic measure. A 2009 study by psychology researchers at the University College London indicates that it takes on average sixty-six days to create a habit. The number of subjects in the study was quite small. But the findings do suggest that it takes at the very least a couple of months of intense effort to create a habit and may even take up to a year for it to fully automate and integrate into a lifestyle.[16] Naturally, some behaviors become habituated more quickly than others.

Finally, after some time, the truth I had learned began to settle in as an integral part of my walk with God and transformed my thinking and practice of forgiveness. In essence, with the help of a good teacher and God's Spirit, I had formed a new habit and weakened a bad one. My brain was being rewired, stimulating growth into the image of Christ. The negative neural networks were dying . . . to the glory of God.

My obedience reintegrates my life and brings it into better alignment with God's truth. There are still times when I must do intense battle with my thoughts and emotions to honestly forgive someone who has hurt me. But little by little a forgiving spirit becomes a habitual part of who I am and the way I live my life (Level V: Recall with Habit—"I do with consistency"). The prompt to forgive comes more automatically.

In the following chapter we describe further how to build or change daily habits.

SUGGESTED LEARNING TASKS

- Encourage people to examine their daily habits before God and identify what he is calling them to change.

- Remind learners that they have the power to change a habit by identifying the cue, the routine, and the reward. Then, using the same cue, begin to change the behavior routine.

- If they want to build a new habit, it is most helpful to connect it to another well-formed habit and use that original habit as a cue to add the new behavior routine.

- Encourage learners wishing to change or build a habit to reach out to others in their small groups for support, problem solving, and prayer.

Finally, remind them to be persistent because persistence helps build consistency. Consistency is fundamental to habit.

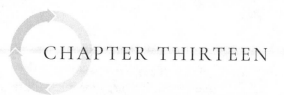

CHAPTER THIRTEEN

Sustaining a Habit

Blessed is the man who perseveres under trial because, having stood the test, that person will receive the crown of life that the Lord has promised to those who love him.

JAMES 1:12

Moreover, it is required of stewards that they be found faithful.

1 CORINTHIANS 4:2 (ESV)

You are what you repeatedly do. Therefore, excellence ought to be a habit not an act.

ARISTOTLE

B EYOND THE BASIC ELEMENTS of habit formation (the cue, the routine, and the reward), researchers are discovering two other elements that work to our advantage. These two elements contribute to sustainability of a new habit, especially those habits that are most difficult to form. These two elements are *belief* and *community.*

THE POWER OF BELIEF

Some particularly obstinate habits like addictions will require more than a simple change in routines or patterns of behavior. Research demonstrates that addressing these habits requires an act of belief. The question is, belief in what?

As noted earlier, Alcoholics Anonymous (AA) is widely known for its success as an alcohol addiction recovery program. It has been so successful that the same approach is used for many other addictions such as cocaine, gambling, and several others including eating disorders. At the core of the AA approach are frequent group meetings and the AA twelve steps to recovery. Six of the twelve AA steps urge the alcoholic to believe that "God" or a "higher power" can help.[1]

Those researching habit determined the belief that the person could succeed was the important element. But alcoholics themselves in their interviews said that when tempted to fall back into old alcoholic patterns, the difference between success and failure was belief in God.

Duhigg explains, "Researchers hated that explanation. God and spirituality are not testable hypotheses. Churches are filled with drunks who continue drinking despite a pious faith."[2]

So a group of researchers from UC Berkeley, Brown University, and the National Institutes of Health started talking with alcoholics about spiritual things. They found that alcoholics who practiced good habit formation techniques were able to stay sober until some stressful event entered their lives and then a "number" relapsed. Those alcoholics, however, who believed that some "higher power" was present in their lives were "more likely" to stay sober.[3]

This same group of researchers determined,

> It wasn't God that mattered. . . . It was belief itself that made a difference. Once people learned how to believe in something, that skill started spilling over to other parts of their lives, until they started believing they could change. Belief was the ingredient that made a reworked habit loop into a permanent behavior.[4]

From a supernatural perspective, Christians believe it *was* God that mattered to the alcoholics' recovery as well as the belief that they were capable of personal change. Both empowered them to rework and build permanent behavior patterns. As children of God we can recall, believe, and celebrate Hebrews 13:6, "So we say with confidence, 'The Lord is my helper; I will not be afraid.'"

The findings show that when tempted to relapse into alcohol use, alcoholics credited God for their strength to stay sober.[5] Human beings are more than just a set of habits, a bunch of neurons stimulated by dopamine. There is more than the physiological reward system. All of this is true and explains in part our decisions and behaviors. But "the more" is based upon the fact that God loves us, cares about us, and is "an ever-present help in trouble" (Ps 46:1).

Hebrews 11 lists people who did unusual things because they believed God would act on what he promised. The Old Testament character Job, under enormous duress, said, "Though He slay me, yet will I trust Him" (Job 13:15 NKJV). All but one of the disciples were martyred for their belief in Jesus Christ. In every generation, down through the ages, Christians have gone willingly to death—burned at the stake, beheaded, and enduring unthinkable persecution—because they knew and believed God, took him at his word, and refused to recant. When we truly believe God is present and working in our situation, we have the courage to do what is right.

KEYSTONE HABITS

Genuine belief in God's help illustrates what researchers call a "keystone habit."[6] When a keystone habit begins to change behavior in one area, known as a "small win," it sets in motion a force that promotes changes in other habitual patterns.[7] According to Duhigg, it can eventually "transform everything."[8] We suggest that the habit of believing in God's help in one specific area—a small win—fosters the belief that personal change is actually possible: another small win. These small wins create a "culture" where change become "contagious."[9]

> *No matter how many times you stumble and fail to achieve victory over your passions do not despair. Every effort you make . . . increases the prospect of eventual victory.*
>
> LEO TOLSTOY, *PATH OF LIFE*

One of my good friends, Judy, has battled pancreatic cancer for over three years. Now her cancer medication seems to be failing her. Providentially, Italian scientists recently produced a new drug with cancer-fighting promise. But several months have slipped away before the medication could be distributed to patients in the United States. Judy has a card posted above her kitchen sink that reminds her of God's presence. She tells me that she sees that card many times each day and is reminded of God's care for her during this difficult period of waiting. The card (a deliberate cue), reminds her of her sovereign God and care for her (a keystone habit routine) that sustains her faith in God, providing hope and preventing a descent into depression and despair (her reward). Judy's new habit is a picture of a thought habit. These habits are not necessarily seen by others unless they are shared. Nevertheless, God-honoring thought habits can have a great deal of power over our lives.

Repetition, also called "rote rehearsal" in the literature, is most useful for committing important information to memory: a Scripture verse, a poem, a song, the multiplication tables, or anything necessary for exact and longer-term recall.[10] Much of repetition is used for memorizing data for a test. When Judy reminded herself of God's presence and care (keystone habit), she was also relying on repetition to imprint that truth deep in her long-term memory for present and later use.

One of my keystone habits. Several years ago, I experienced the power of belief in God's help to change. Quite unexpectedly, I formed a simple but permanent thought habit (keystone habit). I was working for the international division of World Relief. I desperately needed to believe that God would help me and give me wisdom to solve some problems in a difficult situation.

I was traveling in Bangladesh and encountered God's help in a way that still warms my heart as I think about it. New in the position as the director of child survival for World Relief, I traveled for the first time to our child survival program in Khulna, deep in the rural regions of Bangladesh. Several major problems plagued this massive program designed to train some eighty thousand mothers to keep their children alive until they reached the less vulnerable age of six.

There was much I still needed to learn. I had no one to fall back on for advice about the problems I was expected to solve. Beyond the difficulties in the program, upon arrival at the Dhaka airport, I felt a darkness descend on my spirit—a sense of depression that just hung over me like a cloud refusing to lift.

After a restless hot night in the Kuhlna guest house, at dawn I knelt by my bed, poured out my angst to God, begging him to help me make it through the day. As I finished praying, I heard a strange little repetitive sound, "tck, tck, tck," like a marble hitting a pane of glass. I looked around for the source of the "tck, tck, tck" and finally identified it as coming from a couple of little geckos crawling the wall. Immediately I sensed God saying to me, "I'm here just like those geckos. I made them. They belong to me. Let them remind you of me. I'll go with you and help you today." Then a gecko cried again—"tck, tck, tck."

I went to breakfast and heard the same "tck, tck, tck" from another gecko on the wall. I sensed God's presence wash over me once more. And so, a new cue, a new thought routine, and the beautiful reward of knowing God was present was launched in my life. For the next two and a half weeks in Bangladesh, through all the meetings and thorny discussions, several times each day, the geckos would make their familiar sound and God's presence and belief in his help would comfort me. Each day this little gecko's cry was a cue that elicited the same thought routine: reminding me that God was present—helping me and giving me confidence as I worked through the problems. I'd like to say that all the problems were solved by the time I left, but that isn't exactly true. However, I had the confidence to suggest solutions to some of the issues and left feeling that my time there achieved what God intended. Unresolved issues would keep for the next trip.

> *Belief is an essential brain changer; without it, your brain will not provide the resources required to accomplish whatever is in your sights.*
>
> DAVID DiSALVO, *BRAIN CHANGER*

Admittedly, this was a strange little habit that formed when least expected and most needed. It cemented itself into my brain, augmented by the belief that God was present and ready to help. Not only that, but every time, years later, upon returning to Bangladesh or Asia, the gecko cry precipitated that beautiful thought routine all over again, along with the feeling of joy in knowing God was there and willing to help.

KEYSTONE HABITS AND STARTER HABITS

Keystone habits can also function as starter habits. Starter habits provide the small wins that dovetail with the larger, more important habits making change contagious. When Duane was in elementary school, he had the bad habit of biting his fingernails. His repeated failures to stop discouraged him terribly because of the embarrassment it caused. Then he stumbled on the idea of not biting one nail . . . the one he used to point, his index finger. He could hide his embarrassment most of the time. He felt so good (reward), he stopped biting a second (reward). Soon a third was added and then he quit altogether never to return to that nasty habit. Small, doable steps (small wins) carried him to victory.

The book *The 5 Second Rule* by Mel Robbins identifies a starter habit designed to overcome the typical debate that rages in our brains once we are prompted to do what we know we should do (the cue) but don't feel like it. Robbins discovered her five-second rule during a dark, depressive period in her life characterized by total inaction. Reluctant to face her massive problems, she would hit the snooze button over and over in the morning to the point where she had become incapable of managing her day, let alone her life.

One night she watched a NASA rocket launch on TV. As the engineers counted the seconds down, "five, four, three, two, one, blastoff," it hit her. She could use the countdown to launch herself out of bed in the morning. The next morning when the alarm sounded, she counted, "five, four, three, two, one, blastoff," and climbed out of bed. The launch count distracted her brain from listing all the reasons to hit the snooze button. Robbins initiated this starter habit to begin several other important habits that eventually turned her life around. Since then, her book *The 5 Second Rule* has inspired her myriads of readers to use this little habit to launch many other life-changing habits. Employing the five-second rule blocks the brain's desire to procrastinate, especially if the new habit implies difficulty. Robbins warns the reader against counting forward because it is too easy just to keep counting and never act.[11]

THE POWER OF SUPPORT GROUPS

The first element that contributes to habit sustainability is belief. A second element contributing to sustainable habit formation is community, belonging to a supportive group. Not all behavior change requires a support group, but by all means do not minimize its value. An empathic group actually bolsters a person's belief that change is possible; so the two elements, belief and a support group, function as mutual reinforcers. The group may be as small as just two people.

Alcoholics Anonymous groups. AA groups are based on a "peer group model," meaning that the alcoholic learns that he or she doesn't have all the answers, that it is okay to ask for help and to learn from each other."[12]

We, the authors, contend that the best learning often happens within a supportive group. If the content is important, then working to change our habits and integrating that content into our lifestyle will often require a group of caring, praying people. Mezirow's theory of transformative learning also shows the importance of learning communities or support groups. We need the wisdom of a group—people on the same journey—for courage, confidence, counsel, caution, and celebration.

Lee Ann Kaskutas, a senior scientist at the Alcohol Research Group writes,

> At some point, people in AA look around the room and think, *if it worked for that guy, I guess it can work for me.* There's something really powerful about groups and shared experiences. People might be skeptical about their ability to change if they're by themselves, but a group will convince them to suspend disbelief. A community creates belief.[13]

Mirror neurons. Of interest to the discussion of support groups are the brain findings on "mirror neurons." It would appear that some of the power of support groups to influence how we act is due to mirror neurons. Early fMRI technology noticed mirror neurons in monkeys, which seemed to explain certain behaviors. When a monkey performed a certain behavior, a set of neurons fired in the brain of an observing monkey just prior to mimicking the same behavior. "Monkey see, monkey do" may illustrate. Observing an action of the experimenter generated a similar action in the observing monkey—again, the action of mirror neurons firing just prior to the action. Eventually the same phenomenon was observed in humans.

> [Mirror neurons] allow us to recreate the experiences of others within ourselves and to understand others' emotions and empathize. Seeing the look of disgust or joy on other people's faces causes mirror neurons to trigger similar emotions in us. We start to feel their actions and sensations as though we were doing them.[14]

Behaviors of people around us tend to influence us as our behaviors tend to influence them. People sharing stimulates neural activity, which tends to be contagious. It prompts other people to do the same. So the group members feel and share both the content of the discussions as well as the emotions behind the content. Our own observations of watching people in dyads or small groups validate the richness of what transpires as people enter learning together.

The complexity of the brain, however, cautions everyone not to overstate premises. Eyler warns that researchers may be inflating the influence of mirror neurons, declaring that they are not the "holy grail in terms of unlocking the

secrets of the human mind."[15] Thus, as we noted early in this book, we have
tried to reference the brain research that has been stable over the years and
provide reasonable application to our vocation of teaching, mentoring, nurturing. The study of mirror neurons has been prominent in the literature, and
we offer our measured interpre-
tation and application cautiously.

*The church "has put
too much faith in the
use of words and used
too little the language
of relationship."*

REUEL HOWE, *THE
MIRACLE OF DIALOGUE*

Saddleback Church groups. Besides AA, Duhigg cites a second example, demonstrating the power of
a group to contribute to the formation of new behavior habits. This
story comes from Rick Warren's
hugely successful Saddleback
church in Orange, California. Now
forty years old, the church has twenty-five thousand parishioners and fifteen
satellites with thousands of other churches based on the Saddleback model.[16]

Duhigg states, "At the core of his church's growth and [Warren's] success
is a fundamental belief in the power of social habits."[17] He explains that
Warren, as a seminary student, was challenged by Donald McGavran's writing
on how to plant churches in unchurched areas. McGavran held that church
planters should endeavor to bring groups of people to Christ so as not to
destroy their existing social relationships, which he termed "social habits." It
is widely accepted that most successful movements like the civil rights
movement succeeded in part because they depended on social networks to
create new "social habits" (McGavran's term). McGavran's premise was that
new Christians would find it easier to develop the life habits if they were
developed within a social context. Warren took this advice. At Saddleback,
Warren nurtures the formation of spiritual disciplines, or "habits of faith,"
within an organized system of neighborhood groups.

HABITS OF FAITH

In an interview Warren said,

> We've thought long and hard about habitualizing faith, breaking it down into
> pieces. . . . If you try to scare people into following Christ's example, it's not
> going to work for too long. The only way you get people to take responsibility
> for their spiritual maturity is to teach them *habits* of faith."[18]

Now, thirty-five years later, his church offers a curriculum for each of the four habits of faith in the small groups. The four habits are daily time in the Bible, prayer, giving, and fellowship.[19] Together in their weekly group, neighbors work though these curricula and build into their lives these four transformative habits. Alcoholics Anonymous and the example of Saddleback church affirm the power a group of people can have to change minds and create new habits that yield transformed lives.

So how do you create a habit or replace a bad habit? Choose a cue, determine the routine, and ask yourself what reward would motivate the formation of this habit.

A while back, Duane pointed out that I have a bad driving habit—my tendency to drive closer to the center line rather than hug the safer right side. He was right. Upon consideration, I knew what my new routine should be: to drive closer to the right of the lane. However, the question remained, *what cue and what reward would ensure that the habit would stick?* One day while driving together with my eleven-year-old granddaughter, I explained my dilemma and asked her to suggest a reward.

> *Faith, hope, love, and the ninefold fruit are things which demand to be practiced, learned, and made habitual together.*
>
> N. T. WRIGHT, *AFTER YOU BELIEVE*

She thought that having Grandpa pay me five dollars each time I followed the rule would work. After some discussion she agreed that perhaps it would be better if the reward were reduced to twenty-five cents. But I knew that a more relaxed husband at my side while I was driving would be sufficient reward for me. However, the cue remained a problem for me. My driving after all these years is almost completely automatic. My practical granddaughter did suggest that I could place a sticky note on the dash or the steering wheel until the better driving habit was established. Perhaps that will be sufficient. The point is we need to identify our own cues, routines, and rewards that will work for us.

THE OUTLIER PHARISEE

Jesus used a very confrontational and provocative tone in addressing the hypocrisy of the Pharisees and teachers of the law (Mt 23; see chapter 2). They did not practice what they taught.

There was, however, an outlier named Nicodemus, also a Pharisee and a member of the "Jewish ruling council" (Jn 3:1). Nicodemus was like the other Pharisees in that he, too, knew the Old Testament well (Recall). But unlike most of the Pharisees he made different choices. He remained open, conversed extensively with Jesus (Jn 3:2-15) and eventually affirmed his emerging beliefs. Nicodemus was curious about Jesus' teaching and found value and relevance for his life choices (Recall with Appreciation). Jesus told Nicodemus that he (Jesus) would be lifted up like the snake Moses raised in the wilderness so that "everyone who believes may have eternal life in him" (Jn 3:15).

Obviously, Nicodemus must then have pondered the implications of Jesus—his person and teaching (Recall with Speculation) and made a decision to become a follower of Jesus, albeit a secret follower. Even so, he faced daunting *barriers* (Jn 7:50-52). At Jesus' trial he asked the simple question, "Does our law condemn a man without first hearing him to find out what he has been doing?" The Pharisees' disapproval was swift and personal, "Are you from Galilee too?" Clearly Nicodemus was beginning to act on his beliefs (Recall with Practice). In the end, we see his strong commitment to Jesus as he helps Joseph of Arimathea prepare Jesus' body for burial (Jn 19:39). This Pharisee had transformed his perspective and made the risky choice to act on his belief. We hear no more about him in Scripture, but trust that he went on to make living for Christ a lifelong habit (Recall with Habit).

Like Nicodemus, we do well to be outliers as we follow Jesus. May we remember truth, value it, think about how it affects our practices and make the changes knowing the barriers we face. Finally, let us build habits that reflect the character of our God as seen in Jesus.

As we think about establishing better habits, small or large, we need to grasp the basic cue, routine, and reward. But beyond that, we must consider the power of belief—belief that the routine is right and good and that God will help us change. Then we find others who are taking the same journey to pilgrim with as we commit to that new habit.

The end of any significant learning event is being able to glimpse a truth-based habit as it settles into a learner's lifestyle, be it a daily habit of forgiveness, gratefulness, or God consciousness or the wisdom to solve troublesome human and societal problems. Each positive habit advances the good and contributes to our welfare. Learners are now *inclined* toward what is right and good.

James K. A. Smith sums it up in his book, *You Are What You Love,* "In short, if you are what you love, and love is a habit, then discipleship is a re-habituation of your loves. This means that discipleship is more a matter of *reform*ation than of acquiring *in*formation."[20]

TEACHER'S ROLE SUMMARY

It should be obvious that educators continue to have an important role helping the learners to journey through the entire transformation process from the first exposure to the content (Level I: Recall—"I remember the information") to the development of critical life habits that are established and integrated (Level V: Recall with Habit—"I do consistently"). The educator's role lessens in time as the learners take on more and more responsibility for their own habitual ways of thinking, feeling, and acting.

Suggested ways to assist the learner navigate Level V: Recall with Habit are these:

- Clearly present and reiterate how habits are formed or replaced and help learners personalize the cues, routines, and rewards for whatever changes they hope to make.

- Discuss keystone or starter habits with the learners and encourage them to think of starter habits to launch their new habits.

- Create a support group of likeminded learners where they can discuss successes and failures in a safe environment and make plans to overcome the barriers they are encountering.

- Create open questions that stimulate reflection on changes the learners are hoping to achieve, their thinking about how well they are doing, and what barriers they are encountering in their attempts to change their habits.

- Regularly rehearse the content (Recall), driving the transformation in order to solidify it in the learners' long-term memory and heighten the likelihood that the truth will create sustainable life transformation.

Acknowledge the importance of believing in God's help. Spend time in prayer, asking for God's help and intervention in each personal transformation.

The Learning Cycle

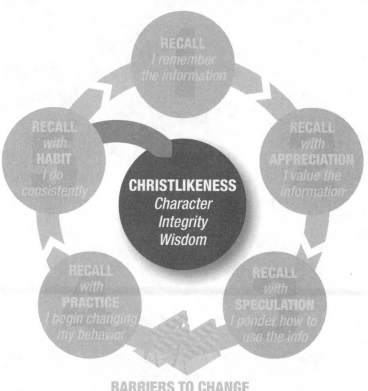

RECALL
I remember
the information

RECALL
with
APPRECIATION
I value the
information

RECALL
with
HABIT
I do
consistently

CHRISTLIKENESS
Character
Integrity
Wisdom

RECALL
with
PRACTICE
I begin changing
my behavior

RECALL
with
SPECULATION
I ponder how to
use the info

BARRIERS TO CHANGE

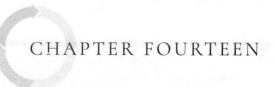

CHAPTER FOURTEEN

From Habit to Character

But we must never forget that Jesus points beyond action to the source of action in character. This is a general principle that governs all he says.

DALLAS WILLARD, *THE DIVINE CONSPIRACY*

To know truth we must follow it with our lives.

PARKER PALMER, *TO KNOW AS WE ARE KNOWN*

Being confident of this, that he who began a good work in you will carry it on to completion until the day of Christ Jesus.

PHILIPPIANS 1:6

GOD HAS GIVEN PEOPLE TRUTH through the Holy Scriptures and through his creation. His purpose in doing this was that his followers, "dead in [their] transgressions and sins," could be saved from their sinful state and be transformed into the image of Christ (Eph 2:1). *Knowing, believing, doing, and being the truth* would be the means by which all of this would happen. In so doing, his followers would act as vice regents over all of his creation, revealing the Creator's love and saving power as well as promoting justice and compassion.

Believers are called to be redemptive agents working to bring all things back under the authority of God. In this sense, we pray, "thy kingdom come." Believers are about the restoration of God's kingdom rule on earth—back to what God originally intended. Being worthy vice regents assumes we know, believe, and live in ways that reflect the values of the King. Jesus showed us the way.

BACK TO THE BEGINNING

This book attempts to set forth a way in which knowledge of the truth can be the beginning of a process whereby people (1) remember truth, (2) value truth, (3) commit to doing truth, (4) overcome obstacles, (5) begin acting upon truth, and (6) make truth a sustainable habit in daily life.

This pattern eventually yields a character, an integrity, a wisdom that reveals the One who said, "I am . . . the truth" (Jn 14:6). Only when all of these steps are transacted can we say we have educated. And, by the way, we are all educators. Jan Hábl in his insightful treatise of Comenius states,

> For what is knowledge without morality? . . . He who makes progress in knowledge but not in morality . . . recedes rather than advances. . . . Therefore, an education that was not held together by the "unbreakable bonds" of morality and piety, would be an "unhappy" education.[1] In order that "humanity not fall into inhumanity," Comenius declares, educators must teach people to be knowledgeable, ethical, and to "turn to God, the source of everything."[2]

Dallas Willard commented on the state of Christianity,

> Whatever the ultimate explanation of it, the most telling thing about the contemporary Christian is that he or she simply has no compelling sense that understanding of and conformity with the clear teachings of Christ is of any vital importance to his or her life, and certainly not that it is in any way essential.[3]

The authors have made an attempt to address the problem Willard poses by suggesting a model—a teaching-learning model that can be seen as journey—for it is a lifetime effort culminated by Christ's return when we become "like him, for we shall see him as he is" (1 Jn 3:2).

THE JOURNEY IN BRIEF

Chapters one and two: God has given us all we need to be transformed and to be his agents of transformation in this world. But the problem of the religious leaders of Jesus' day is our problem: knowing the Word but living as though it was irrelevant or optional, otherwise known as hypocrisy. Living a more integrated life is not only possible but necessary to honor God and fulfill his purposes for us and for the church. To achieve this ambitious goal, educators, parents, pastors—all who provide nurture—must shoulder the burden, yea, the privilege. To be sure, there are challenges and many of us have a natural resistance to change.

Chapters three and four: Building a biblical knowledge base as foundation for the Christian faith has always been a strength of evangelical institutions. If knowing and doing were inseparable, it could be a more ideal world: what we teach is exactly what is learned and lived. However, in the transition from *knowing* Scripture to *doing* it, the *doing it* remains the weaker partner. But it doesn't need to stay that way.

Chapter five: Valuing truth and embracing it emanates from a positive response to knowledge. The brain research conclusively states that positive emotions open the way for the rational, thinking, logical part of the brain to function. Therefore, a knowledge that leads to obedience is unlikely unless acknowledging and building positive affect (emotions) are an intentional part of the teaching.

Chapters six and seven: Speculation is the nexus between the classroom (or wherever you teach) and life. Failure to provide time for learners to reflect on the "So what should I do with this truth I value?" question allows that truth to lie in a vacuum soon to be lost from short-term memory. Speculation takes the learner into the realm of what should be and opens the potential truth to become part of working memory and, eventually, long-term memory—where it influences the practice of truth.

Chapters eight and nine: Anytime someone determines to live a more obedient life, there will be barriers. Some are internal or personal, some social, some cultural. To be aware of potential barriers and to have an action plan advances the likelihood the decision will be realized. Space in the learning environment and an invitation to others to join in this difficult part of the journey are necessary components for success.

Chapters ten and eleven: Until now, obedience has been largely an activity of the mind and affect (emotion or valuing)—relatively easy but absolutely necessary. The early *practice* of the truth must be carefully thought out and acted upon because failure can be devastating if not permanent. Teachers, mentors, parents, peers amplify in importance at this level.

Chapters twelve and thirteen: Continuous practice of the obedience God has prompted and the Holy Spirit has empowered eventually takes the form of habit. Obeying becomes an act of love and devotion rather than duty. Obedience matures from "what I should do" to "what I want to do" because that is who I am and what I want to be in relation to my magnificent God. Life becomes more integral, more whole. Each virtue that is forged into my character honors the God who prompts that virtue. And he finds joy in seeing it expressed in his people. Besides integrity and character, we get wisdom, which is living according to God's truth. Perhaps that is why Solomon proclaimed that wisdom is supreme (see Prov 4:7).

THE LEARNING CYCLE APPLIED

Applied to a group of pastors in China: Earlier we talked about our ministry with a group of Chinese pastors who at first were reluctant to discuss but soon participated with enthusiasm. Here is the rest of the story. Another group of similar size to ours, also pastors, was in a nearby classroom where a world class author and lecturer was teaching. As we closed the week, everyone from both groups gathered in a large room seated in a circle. Our host asked the group, "Let's take a few minutes to share one specific thing we learned this week and how it will help our ministry." One person popped up immediately and answered. She was from our group. Another stood. Same story, from our group. This was repeated seven or eight times. The host stepped in and asked to hear from someone from the other group. After fifteen or twenty seconds of silence one person slowly stood and said: "We learned many things this week and I'm sure some will be useful in the future."

The content in the other class was excellent because we knew the teacher. But it would seem the content (Recall) remained mostly in their notes. We failed to observe any sense of personal relevance (Recall and Appreciation) nor any evidence of potential application (Recall and Speculation) for ministry.

Applied to an institution in Bulgaria: Nik stood at a gathering of about twenty European theological educators. His words thundered the conclusion of the hour-long discussion: "We have imported the best of theological education from the West and it has not done the job for us." Nik soon invited GATE (Global Associates for Transformational Education—see chapter 11) to come to Bulgaria and do a workshop for four faculties and administrators. Three days each year for four years GATE personnel asked questions, facilitated discussion, provided some content and set aside space for individuals and faculties to reflect, to determine priorities and set goals. The following year the goals were debriefed and the process continued.

Last week, in Sofia, I talked with Nik, now retired but still active, and he told me: "Almost the entire faculty changed their teaching style because of the four years GATE invested in us, and we believe the students are better equipped than before. Thank you." Scores of faculties in Europe, Asia, Africa, and South America have been similarly influenced.

Applied to an individual, Ron: He sat in my (Duane's) human development class. Always in the back row and in the corner, he was not the most respectful student. He had a reputation for being more interested in things other than learning. His frequent whispering and laughing brought looks from me that I hoped would discourage his distracting behavior. His assignments were done well and showed an astute mind. About halfway into the semester I had finished a teaching section on moral reasoning/knowledge (Recall) and moral behavior (Recall with Practice), essentially the Pharisees' issue. It would appear Ron experienced some dissonance between his belief system and his behavior choices. He now realized they were in contradiction.

Ron had been raised in a Christian home and knew the Scriptures, but now he was confronted with the gap between his knowing and doing. Because he valued (emotion) his faith and had no desire to forfeit his beliefs, he now arrived at a crossroads: Which to choose? Ron chose the way of obedience (Speculation). Yes, there were bumps (barriers) along the way. But Ron persevered, changed, and saw his habits of faith fuse into a person of character, integrity, and wisdom. Today he enjoys regional leadership in his denomination, pastors a local church, has a growing international ministry, and finds great satisfaction in his family, all of whom share in his journey of obedience. The highest honor we personally can pay to Ron is that when we have problems we need help with, he is one of the first people we call. Enough said.

CHANGE IS HARD

Anyone who has tried to keep a New Year's resolution knows sustainable change requires enormous perseverance. Educators Bowen and Watson write, "Neurologists, developmental psychologists, organizational business gurus, residential life professionals, therapists, and educational theorists have all come to the same conclusion: change is hard, and it requires motivation, persistence, design, and support."[4]

The Learning Cycle model (chapters four through fourteen) was crafted to help educators design their classes, motivate their learners, create support among peers, and aid in persistence (self-discipline) to enact truth in one's life. At each stage of the Learning Cycle we have tried to offer learning tasks we have used and found effective: case studies, problem solving, one-on-one dialogue, group discussion, open questions, reflection, speculation, memos to myself, field experiences, instructional simulations, biographies, video clips, and others.

When learning tasks are added to content delivery (lectures) in appropriate time segments, learning can be exponential. Most activities engaging the student's mind and emotions become more memorable and more likely to enter working and long-term memory. Only when stored in long-term memory do beliefs and behavior begin the fusion into integrity, character, and wisdom. This we call Christlikeness.

Anything worth doing usually demands attention and work over multiple time frames. Furthermore, Christians recognize there is an adversary who would seek to undermine if not destroy the character, integrity, and wisdom we seek. It is well to remember that we have been given armor with which to fight (Rom 13:11-14; 2 Cor 6:7; Eph 6:10-20; 1 Pet 4:1-2). Additionally the Holy Spirit is our guide in leading us to truth, and the power of the resurrected Christ gives hope in the ultimate victory.

CHARACTER, INTEGRITY AND WISDOM

Character determines how knowledge is used. As Plato noted, "Knowing becomes evil if the aim be not virtuous." Thus, *character*, *integrity*, and *wisdom* matter. We have chosen these three words to form a capstone for the Learning Cycle. These three are not the only words that might be placed in the center of learning. If we were to choose only one word it would be "Christlikeness." The final goal boils down to looking and being like Jesus.

N. T. Wright offers sound reasoning on becoming that transformed person. Using Paul's clothing metaphor in Colossians 3, Wright states,

> As with the "putting off," so the "putting on" is a matter of consciously deciding, again and again, to do certain things in certain ways, to create patterns of memory and imagination deep within the psyche and, as we saw from contemporary neuroscience, deep within the actual physical structure of our mysterious brain. Gradually, bit by bit, the "putting on" of these qualities—qualities

that seem for the moment so artificial, so unnatural, so "unlike me"—will in fact transform the character at its deepest level.[5]

Colossians 3:12-17 provides the Christian with list of virtues to "put on." They will feel unnatural, even artificial, if they are new to us. But with time, the unnatural becomes natural, even preferred, because these virtues draw us closer to the image of Christ. An excellent discipline is to study the list regularly as a reminder of what we are to "put on" each morning. Paul summarizes: "And over all these virtues put on love, which binds them all together in perfect unity" (Col 3:14).[6]

Wright continues,

> *Intelligence plus character—that is the goal of education.*
>
> MARTIN LUTHER KING JR.

When Paul talks about the "mind," he is not ranking Christians in terms of what we could call their intellectual or "academic" ability. . . . Paul wants all Christians to have their minds renewed, so that they can think *in a different way*. . . . We have to be able to think about what to do—what to do with our whole lives. . . . Being trained to think Christianly is the antidote to what will otherwise happen: being, as Paul says, "squeezed into the shape dictated by the present age.[7]

[The] renewal of the mind is at the center of the renewal of the whole human being, since the "darkening" of the mind we identified as central to the problem of idolatry, dehumanization, and sin in an earlier chapter of Romans (1:2-23, 28).[8]

Change requires discipline, perseverance, and support from others—all bathed in prayer—because obedience is worth it. Some things you just must go after. Waiting for them to happen constitutes failure. Thomas A. Huxley, British biologist and educator, said, "The great end of life is not knowledge, but action."

This seems to be the message of Matthew 7:24-27. Keep in mind the

> *To know and not to do is to not yet know.*
>
> KURT LEWIN

context is "who will enter the kingdom of heaven" and who will hear, "I never knew you" (Mt 7:21-23). The significant difference between the wise and foolish person is that one hears "these words of mine" and "puts them into practice;" the other hears but does not "put them into practice" (Mt 7:24, 26). So who "will enter the kingdom of heaven"? "Only the one who does the will of my Father who is in heaven" (Mt 7:21).

CAUTION REGARDING IMBALANCE

One good side effect of the Learning Cycle is that we see more clearly where we can improve our teaching and nurturing. Most of us are strong on the knowing (or content), but we also must consider our ability to (1) build positive affect, (2) prompt speculation, (3) identify barriers, (4) support practice, and (5) help establish habits.

Some unintended side effects may occur:

- Overemphasis on recall or remembering can incline people toward *hypocrisy*.

- Overemphasis on valuing or emotion can incline people toward *instability*.

- Overemphasis on barriers or obstacles can incline people toward *paralysis*.

- Overemphasis on speculation or transfer can incline people toward *inaction*.

- Overemphasis on practice or changing can incline people toward unreflective *activism*.

- Overemphasis on habit or consistency can incline people toward empty *routine*.

None of these five levels of our Learning Cycle stands alone, a weakness of many models. When each is present in the learning environment, they become mutually reinforcing and each plays both a distinct and integrative role. Overlook emotion, and content tends to be forgotten. Eliminate speculation or transfer, and learners become complacent in the cognitive (remembering), believing that obedience is optional. All are necessary for the goal of a faithful life.

CONTINUE THE LEARNING

It appears the Learning Cycle is a closed system. So what happens to future learning? To respond, it is helpful to think of the Learning Cycle as a spiral ever expanding its way upward. To explain that, at least in part, takes us back to cognitive dissonance. In a learning task, when learners engage truth and put it into practice, new questions often arise, suggesting new insights to explore, new applications to pursue. This inspires a need for new knowledge to shed light and discover truth as best as it can be attained. The brain loves to solve problems, to reason, to struggle, to find answers—to work.[9] Dissonance is another way of saying there is a problem to be solved, a disconnect that needs understanding, a situation that needs insight, a decision that must be carefully thought through. It is not always dissonance that prompts thought and change; it can be curiosity, a simple conversation, reading a book, or just a growing concern that you need to do something different—and so the Learning Cycle begins anew.

As the learner completes the cycle by making some behavior habitual, there will be "space" to engage new challenges created by life experiences in whatever form they may take, from casual discussions with others, to challenges at work or in the family, to crises that need a response.

When confronted with life situations we are driven back to "Recall": What does God say about how we should manage this moment? What biblical or creational truth can I glean for guidance? Do I sense a guidance or conviction (emotion) from the Holy Spirit about what is right (value)? What kingdom values are at stake (reflection)? What are the possibilities for action (speculation)? What obstacles will I face (barriers) and how can I plan to handle them? Where do I begin in my response (practice) and what help do I need to be successful? How might this practice become sustainable (habit)? The cycle repeats itself, each time leaving "deposits" in the building of character, integrity, and wisdom—in becoming more Christlike.

In its most succinct form, this book is about teaching for *orthodoxy* (correct knowing or believing), *orthopathos* (appropriate emotions or feelings stemming from correct knowing and believing), and disciplined *orthopraxis* (living truthfully).

We believe it worthwhile to repeat a statement made early in the book. Much of our book assumes Christians teaching in the biblical sciences, but we hope some of our illustrations have alerted those of you in other professions that the model applies in all of formal education as well in the informal nurturing moments of each day. Thus, we have used it with medical workers, community development people, nursing programs, culture sensitivity programs, faculties of colleges and universities, conflict resolution conferences, multinational corporations, theological education conferences, counseling, as well Sunday school classes and pastoral roles.

On a personal note, it has been our privilege to research and write this book. It seemed clear God wanted us to do it. It would not have happened had we made the decision on our own. We hope you have not only enjoyed the journey with us but that your faith has been made more robust, your teaching enriched and your life of obedience inspired.

Join us in affirming the words of Moses, "Everything the LORD has said we will do" (Ex 24:3).

And the words of the Apostle Peter:

> His divine power has given us everything we need for a godly life through our knowledge of him who called us by his own glory and goodness. Through these he has given us his very great and precious promises, so that through them you may participate in the divine nature, having escaped the corruption in the world caused by evil desires. For this very reason, make every effort to add to your faith goodness; and to goodness, knowledge; and to knowledge, self-control; and to self-control, perseverance; and to perseverance, godliness; and to godliness, mutual affection; and to mutual affection, love. For if you possess these qualities in increasing measure, they will keep you from being ineffective and unproductive in your knowledge of the Lord Jesus Christ. (2 Pet 1:3-8)

And Paul encourages us: "And whatever you do, whether in word or deed, do it all in the name of the Lord Jesus, giving thanks to God the Father through him" (Colossians 3:17).

Notes

1. Laying the Foundation

[1] A few years later Moses took his own life. I miss him. The tragic sadness still lingers in my memory.

[2] L. Berkhof, *Systematic Theology* (Grand Rapids, MI: Eerdmans, 1941), 434-35.

[3] Parker Palmer, *The Courage to Teach* (1998; San Francisco: Jossey-Bass, 2007), 68.

[4] B. S. Bloom, ed., *Taxonomy of Educational Objectives, Handbook I: The Cognitive Domain* (New York: Longmans, Green, 1956). D. R. Krathwohl, B. S Bloom, and B. B. Masia, *Taxonomy of Educational Objectives, Handbook II: Affective Domain* (New York: David McKay, 1964). Krathwohl and Bloom did not write a taxonomy of psychomotor (behavioral) objectives, but others did. E. J. Simpson, *The Classification of Educational Objectives in the Psychomotor Domain* (Washington, DC: Gryphon House, 1972).

[5] Recall, Comprehension, Application, Analysis, Synthesis, and Evaluation. *Application* for Bloom usually referred to the mental activity of knowing how or what to do. We use the term to refer to actual *doing*.

[6] David Kolb, *Experiential Learning: Experience as the Source of Learning and Development* (Englewood Cliffs, NJ: Prentice Hall, 1984). Since the more recent findings on the brain and learning, Kolb's model and subsequent updates have come under considerable criticism. Schenck and Cruickshank summarize those critiques and propose a "biological model of teaching" (the Co-Constructed Development Teaching Theory, CDTT) based on neurobiological findings related to experiential learning, which has yet to be tested. The CDTT contains many of the same elements as our Learning Cycle. Jeb Schenck and Jessie Cruickshank, "Evolving Kolb: Experiential Education in the Age of Neuroscience," *Journal of Experiential Education* 38, no.1 (2015): 73-95.

[7] Prochaska's Stages of Change is a psychological behavioral change model that has also been highly researched. This model provides considerable support to our entire Learning Cycle. James O Prochaska, J. C. Prochaska, and John C. Norcross, "Stages of Change," *Psychotherapy* 38, no. 4 (Winter 2001): 443-48.

[8] David A. Sousa, *How the Brain Learns* (Thousand Oaks, CA: Corwin, 2017), 4.

[9] Sousa, *How the Brain Learns*, 22.

[10] Sousa, *How the Brain Learns*, 23.

[11] We use the term "neural networks" consistently in this book but the reader will note that some authors use "neural pathways" (Jensen, see ch. 1, note 12) or "neuronal networks"

(Zull, see ch. 3, note 2). In using "neural networks" we are *not* referring to the information technology (IT) use of the term, which refers to the way a computer attempts to mimic the brain functions using algorithms, sometimes called "deep learning."

[12]Eric Jensen, *Teaching with the Brain in Mind,* 2nd ed. (Alexandria, VA: Association for Supervision and Curriculum, 2005), 17. See also, Britt Andreatta, *Wired to Grow: Harness the Power of Brain Science to Master Any Skill* (Santa Barbara, CA: 7th Mind, 2016), 85.

[13]Howard Gardner, foreword to *Emotions, Learning, and the Brain,* by Mary Helen Immordino-Yang (New York: Norton, 2015), 9.

2. WEAVING TRUTH AND LIFE

[1]Land grant universities, such as MSU, were formed by President Lincoln to create knowledge that would address the problems of the local communities—thus, knowledge that informed action to improve living.

[2]For the most part our MSU professors were deeply committed to the scientific method. They believed this methodology was the best way to discover what was true or factual about our world. Since then, university professors seem more driven by a postmodern ideology having largely abandoned the idea of scientific objectivity, at least in the social sciences.

[3]For brevity we will sometimes refer to these two groups, Pharisees and teachers of the law, simply as Pharisees.

[4]Parker Palmer, *A Hidden Wholeness: The Journey Toward an Undivided Life* (San Francisco: Jossey-Bass, 2009), 7.

[5]Lawrence O. Richards, *A Theology of Christian Education* (Grand Rapids, MI: Zondervan, 1975), 71.

[6]James Davison Hunter, *The Death of Character: Moral Education in an Age without Good or Evil* (New York: Basic Books, 2000), xv.

3. RECALL, REHEARSAL, AND RETENTION

[1]For this reason anthropologists insist that field notes be recorded within twenty-four hours to preserve accuracy.

[2]Researchers sometimes refer to long-term memory as long-term potentiation (LTP). See James E. Zull, *From Brain to Mind: Using Neuroscience to Guide Change in Education* (Sterling, VA: Stylus, 2011), 182-83.

[3]Summarized from David A. Sousa, *How the Brain Learns,* 5th ed. (Thousand Oaks, CA: Corwin, 2017), 86-91; and James E. Zull, *The Art of Changing the Brain: Enriching the Practice of Teaching by Exploring the Biology of Learning* (Sterling, VA: Stylus, 2002), 34.

[4]Zull, *Art of Changing the Brain,* 34. James E. Zull is professor of Biology and Biochemistry and Director of the Center for Innovation in Teaching and Education at Case Western Reserve University. This and his other book, *From Brain to Mind,* offer more detailed treatment of the brain and learning.

[5]Sousa, *How the Brain Learns,* 55-57.

[6]Jack Mezirow, *Transformative Dimensions of Adult Learning* (San Francisco: Jossey-Bass, 1991); Jack Mezirow, "Transformative Learning: Theory to Practice," in *New Directions for Adult and Continuing Education* 74 (Summer 1997): *Transformative Learning in Actions: Insights from Practice*, ed. P. Cranton (San Francisco: Jossey-Bass, 1997) 5-12; and Zull, *Brain to Mind*, 78.

[7]Zull, *Art of Changing the Brain*, 98.

[8]Sousa, *How the Brain Learns*, 96.

[9]Sousa, *How the Brain Learns*, 99.

[10]C. S. Lewis, "The Weight of Glory," in *The Essential C. S. Lewis*, ed. Lyle W. Dorsett (New York: Collier, 1988), 369.

4. LECTURES THAT TRANSFORM

[1]Read Jeremiah, Lamentations, and Ezekiel, a series of graphic portrayals of people who forgot God.

[2]See Num 25:2-5; 1 Kings 12:32; 16:32; 22:43; Hos 8:11; 11:2.

[3]Rita Smilkstein, *We're Born to Learn: Using the Brain's Natural Learning Process to Create Today's Curriculum*, 2nd ed. (Thousand Oaks, CA: Corwin, 2011), 158; James E. Zull, *The Art of Changing the Brain: Enriching the Practice of Teaching by Exploring the Biology of Learning* (Sterling, VA: Stylus, 2002), 128-29.

[4]See the later chapter on Recall with Habit.

[5]Reuel Howe, *The Miracle of Dialogue* (Minneapolis, MN: Seabury Press, 1963), 30.

[6]David A. Sousa, *How the Brain Learns*, 5th ed. (Thousand Oaks, CA: Corwin, 2017), 48.

[7]Some examples of learning tasks are embedded in the text of our chapters and sometimes they are listed at the end of a chapter.

[8]Jane Vella, *Taking Learning to Task* (San Francisco: Jossey-Bass, 2000), 8.

[9]David Hoffeld, "Want to Know What Your Brain Does When It Hears a Question?" February 21, 2017. Fast Company, www.fastcompany.com/3068341/want-to-know-what -your-brain-does-when-it-hears-a-question.

[10]Rick Warren, *The Purpose Driven Life. What on Earth Am I Here For?* (Grand Rapids, MI: Zondervan, 2002), 320-22.

[11]There is some variability in the fifteen to seventeen–minute frames.

[12]From David Goodman, president of Entrust. David Goodman, "Teaching Adults: The Agony and the Ecstasy," *Engage* 6, no. 3 (Fall 2017): 3, https://mailchi.mp/f4341f79bfb0 /real-people-real-impact-really-426883?e=0dc3ad6d27.

[13]Eric Jensen, *Teaching with the Brain in Mind*, 2nd ed. (Alexandria, VA: Association for Supervision and Curriculum, 2005), 36-37.

[14]Parker Palmer, *The Courage to Teach: Exploring the Inner Landscape of a Teacher's Life* (San Francisco: Jossey-Bass, 1998), 11.

[15]J. A. Bowen and C. E. Watson, *Teaching Naked Techniques: A Practical Guide to Designing Better Classes* (San Francisco: Jossey-Bass, 2017), 188.

[16]If you wish more help on making lectures effective, google "better lectures" or "motivating lectures" or some variation and plenty of advice appears, mostly from professionals.

[17]Sousa, *How the Brain Learns*, 53.

[18]Fred Paas, Alexander Renkl, and John Sweller, "Cognitive Load Theory and Instructional Design: Recent Developments," *Educational Psychologist* 38, no. 1 (2003): 2, https://doi .org/10.1207/S15326985EP3801_1. Italics original.

[19]Paas, Renkl, and Sweller, "Cognitive Load Theory," 2.

[20]Sousa, *How the Brain Learns*, 53.

[21]Joshua R. Eyler, *How Humans Learn* (Morgantown: West Virginia University Press, 2018), 192; Donald A. Bligh, *What's the Use of Lectures?* (San Francisco: Jossey-Bass, 2000); and Sousa, *How the Brain Learns*, 53.

[22]Charles C. Bonwell and James A. Eison, *Active Learning: Creating Excitement in the Classroom* (Washington, DC: George Washington University, 1991).

[23]Connie Malamed, "What is Cognitive Load?" *The eLearning Coach*, http://theelearning coach.com/learning/what-is-cognitive-load/.

[24]Above material summarized from Linda B. Nilson, *Teaching at Its Best: A Research-Based Resource for College Instructors* (San Francisco: Jossey-Bass, 2006), 94-96.

5. The Role of Emotion in Learning

[1]David A. Sousa, *How the Brain Learns* (Thousand Oaks, CA: Corwin, 2017), 50.

[2]*Emotion* is the most frequently used word in the literature. Note that we will be using it often but will also employ several other synonyms such as *affect, valuing, appreciation*, and similar terms of positive regard.

[3]Eric Jensen, *Teaching with the Brain in Mind*, 2nd ed. (Alexandria, VA: Association for Supervision and Curriculum, 2005), 70.

[4]James E. Zull, *From Brain to Mind: Using Neuroscience to Guide Change in Education* (Sterling, VA: Stylus, 2011), 77.

[5]We used various words to describe positive emotions (above), but here are some negative emotions that may be found in the classroom: boredom, anxiety, fear, pessimism, embarrassment, failure, and others. The range of affect in any given person is quite extensive. Both positive and negative affective states profoundly influence learning.

[6]Mary Helen Immordino-Yang and Matthias Faeth, "The Role of Emotion and Skilled Intuition in Learning," in *Mind, Brain, and Education: Neuroscience Implications for the Classroom*, ed. David A. Sousa (Bloomington, IN: Solution Tree Press, 2010), 69.

[7]Joshua R. Eyler, *How Humans Learn: The Science and Stories Behind Effective College Teaching* (Morgantown: West Virginia University Press, 2018), 115; Zull, *Brain to Mind*, 35-36; and Sousa, *How the Brain Learns*, 84-85, 89-90.

[8]W. E. Vine, *The Expanded Vine's Expository Dictionary of New Testament Words*, John R. Kohlenberger III, ed. (Minneapolis, MN: Bethany House Publishers, 1984), 537.

[9]Vine, *Expanded Vine's Expository Dictionary*, 537.

[10]Immordino-Yang and Faeth, "Role of Emotion," 78; see also, Zull, *Art of Changing the Brain*, 73; Rita Smilkstein, *We're Born to Learn: Using the Brain's Natural Learning Process to Create Today's Curriculum*, 2nd ed. (Thousand Oaks, CA: Corwin, 2011), 82.

[11]Jerome M. Kagan, *Galen's Prophecy* (New York: Basic Books, 1994), 39.

[12]Antonio Damasio, *Descartes' Error* (New York: Harcourt Brace, 1994), 53. Italics added.

[13]Immordino-Yang and Faeth, "The Role of Emotion," 78.

[14]Sousa, *How the Brain Learns*, 50.

[15]Smilkstein, *We're Born to Learn*, 82.

[16]Sousa, *How the Brain Learns*, 50.

[17]This question asks the reader to speculate, the subject of Level III: Recall and Speculation.

[18]Zull, *Brain to Mind*, 135-36; Sousa, *How the Brain Learns*, 59-63; Jensen, *Teaching with the Brain in Mind*, 69.

[19]Smilkstein, 82-85.

[20]To be sure, there are times when one realizes a student needs specialized help. Often they visit the campus counseling center on their own, but they may need encouragement because counseling can remain a stigma for some.

[21]Jensen, *Teaching with the Brain in Mind*, 78. It is even more true today than when Jensen wrote this as further citations reveal.

[22]Zull, *Art of Changing the Brain*, 229.

[23]Zull, *Art of Changing the Brain*, 228.

[24]Zull, *Art of Changing the Brain*, 228-29.

[25]This story is repeated from my book, *Cross-Cultural Servanthood: Serving the World in Christlike Humility* (Downers Grove, IL: InterVarsity Press, 2006), 27-28. Ann Templeton Brownlee, I am told, originated this story. However, I have never seen nor been able to locate the original story. The one above is my rendition. Many other versions exist, usually without any source.

[26]Jensen, *Teaching with the Brain in Mind*, 68.

[27]Eyler, *How Humans Learn*, 115.

6. FROM CONTENT TO EXPERIENCE

[1]Still other writers use "extending the information," "imagining," or "imagine the future" in talking about speculation or transfer.

[2]We have seen classes of forty to sixty use this format but with a leader very skilled in facilitation.

[3]David A. Sousa, *How the Brain Learns* (Thousand Oaks, CA: Corwin, 2017), 169.

[4]Lewis, C. S., "The Weight of Glory," in *The Essential C. S. Lewis,* ed. Lyle W. Dorsett (New York: Collier, 1988). My paraphrase.

[5]James E. Zull, *From Brain to Mind: Using Neuroscience to Guide Change in Education* (Sterling, VA: Stylus, 2011); Sousa, *How the Brain Learns*; Eric Jensen, *Teaching with the Brain in Mind*, 2nd ed. (Alexandria, VA: Association for Supervision and Curriculum, 2005).

[6]Zull, *Brain to Mind*, 30-45.

[7]Zull, *Brain to Mind*, 45-46.

[8]Zull, *Brain to Mind*, 47.

[9]Gallup, "2015 Gallup Student Poll Results," accessed August 17, 2019, https://news.gallup
.com/reports/189926/student-poll-2015-results.aspx.

[10]Sousa, *How the Brain Learns*, 169.

[11]Sousa, *How the Brain Learns*, 169.

[12]Rita Smilkstein, *We're Born to Learn: Using the Brain's Natural Learning Process to Create
Today's Curriculum*, 2nd ed. (Thousand Oaks, CA: Corwin, 2011), 153.

[13]The exact words of a female, halfway through her junior year in high school. She had
attended church and Sunday School all her life with her family.

[14]Zull, *Brain to Mind*, 76.

[15]David Hoffeld, "Want to Know What Your Brain Does When It Hears a Question?"
February 21, 2017. Fast Company, www.fastcompany.com/3068341/want-to-know-what
-your-brain-does-when-it-hears-a-question.

7. The Power of Cognitive Dissonance

[1]Saul McLeod, "Cognitive Dissonance," *Simply Psychology,* February 5, 2018, www.simply
psychology.org/cognitive-dissonance.html#leon.

[2]Many others have borrowed, renamed and utilized the concept suggesting its pervasive
usefulness. Following are a few similar terms: "disorienting dilemma," "intrusive marker
events," "convictional moments," "crises." Piaget's "cognitive dissonance," which he asserts is the motor that drives all human growth, emphasizes cognitive consonance (i.e.,
connectivity) whereas Festinger, largely in agreement with Piaget, emphasizes cognitive
dissonance (i.e., disconnectivity).

[3]See chapter two and Mt 23.

[4]Keise Izuma, "What Happens to the Brain When We Experience Cognitive Dissonance?"
in *SA Mind* 26, 6, 72 (November 2015), www.scientificamerican.com/article/what-happens
-to-the-brain-during-cognitive-dissonance1/.

[5]It should be noted that some people refuse to face dissonant situations as did the Pharisees. Rather than learn and change, they fixate where they are or they change but chose
unfortunate options such as disbelief in God, drugs, or other options. Some fixate at their
present stage of spiritual maturity. Little change is seen over the years.

8. Identifying Barriers

[1]Joseph Luciani, "Why 80 Percent of New Year's Resolutions Fail," December 29, 2015, *U.S.
News & World Report*, https://health.usnews.com/health-news/blogs/eat-run/articles
/2015-12-29/why-80-percent-of-new-years-resolutions-fail.

[2]Luciani, "Why 80 Percent of New Year's Resolutions Fail."

[3]Personal pronouns refer to Muriel in chapters eight through thirteen unless otherwise noted.

[4]Some examples from the barrier analysis literature include Bonnie Kittle, *A Practical Guide
to Conducting a Barrier Analysis*, 2nd ed. (New York, NY: Helen Keller International,

2017), www.fsnnetwork.org/sites/default/files/final_second_edition_practical_guide_to
_conducting_barrier_analysis.pdf; Mark Galley, "What is Barrier Analysis?" Think Reli-
ability Blog, July 21, 2017, https://blog.thinkreliability.com/what-is-barrier-analysis; and
"Barrier Analysis," ChangingMinds.org, accessed August 17, 2019, http://changingminds.
org/disciplines/change_management/diagnosing_change/barrier_analysis.htm.

[5]Ken Robinson, *The Element: How Finding Your Passion Changes Everything* (New York:
Penguin Books, 2009), 132; Icek Ajzen and Dolores Albarracin, "Predicting and
Changing Behavior: A Reasoned Action Approach," in *Prediction and Change of Health
Behavior: Applying the Reasoned Action Approach* (Mahwah, NJ: Lawrence Erlbaum,
2007), 5, www.researchgate.net/publication/261796733_Predicting_and_changing
_behavior_A_reasoned_action_approach.

[6]Ajzen and Albarracin, "Predicting and Changing Behavior," 5.

[7]Ajzen and Albarracin, "Predicting and Changing Behavior," 7. The terms in parentheses
are Ajzen and Albarracin's. Notice that if any one of these five beliefs is weak or nonex-
istent, this creates a barrier to behavior change; such barriers tend to fall into one of the
three barrier categories: personal, social, or cultural.

9. OVERCOMING BARRIERS

[1]Charles Duhigg, *The Power of Habit: Why We Do What We Do in Life and Business* (New
York: Random House, 2014), 144. Duhigg is a recognized expert in how to create good
habits and destroy bad habits. His work is currently cited in much of the recent literature
on habit formation.

[2]For more information on conducting role plays, see Ted Ward, "A Role Play: A Community
Learning Activity," in The Ward Archives, accessed August 17, 2019, www.wardarchives
.org/document-archives/simulation-games-and-role-plays/role-play-community
-learning-activity/.

[3]A helpful book for dealing with negative thinking is William Backus and Marie Chapian,
*Telling Yourself the Truth: Find Your Way Out of Depression, Anxiety, Fear, Anger, and
Other Common Problems by Applying the Principles of Misbelief Therapy* (Bloomington,
MN: Bethany House Publishers, 2000).

10. TRANSFORMATIVE LEARNING

[1]James K. A. Smith, *You Are What You Love: The Spiritual Power of Habit* (Grand Rapids,
MI: Brazos Press, 2016), 21.

[2]Carol S. Dweck, *Mindset: The New Psychology of Success,* updated ed. (New York: Random
House, 2017).

[3]Britt Andreatta, *Wired to Grow: Harness the Power of Brain Science to Master Any Skill*
(Santa Barbara, CA: Seventh Mind, 2016).

[4]Dweck, *Mindset,* 6.

[5]Dweck, *Mindset,* 7.

[6]"Dweck came to see that some students aim at performance goals (fixed mindset), while

others (growth mindset) strive toward learning goals. In the first case, you're working to validate your ability. In the second, you're working to acquire new knowledge or skills." Peter C. Brown, Henry L. Roediger III, and Mark A. McDaniel, *Make It Stick: The Science of Successful Learning* (Cambridge, MA: Belknap Press of Harvard University Press, 2014), 180.

[7]Icek Ajzen and Dolores Albarracin, "Predicting and Changing Behavior: A Reasoned Action Approach," in *Prediction and Change of Health Behavior: Applying the Reasoned Action Approach* (Mahwah, NJ: Lawrence Erlbaum, 2007), 3-21, www.researchgate.net/publication/261796733_Predicting_and_changing_behavior_A_reasoned_action_approach.

[8]"The brain's ability to change with experience is often called *plasticity*." James E. Zull, *From Brain to Mind: Using Neuroscience to Guide Change in Education* (Sterling, VA: Stylus Publishing, 2011), 21.

[9]Phillippa Lally et al., "How Habits Are Formed: Modelling Habit Formation in the Real World," *European Journal of Social Psychology* 40, no. 6 (October 2010): 998-1009.

[10]What happens with each repetition? Every nerve (neuron) consists of three parts: a cell body, dendrites (short branches extending from the cell body), and axons (long fibers), all of which carry the electrical signals within our bodies causing us to function and move. The long fibers (axons), which carry electrical signals to other neurons are covered with a sheath, called myelin, which acts as an insulator for the neuron assuring the effectiveness of the signal as it travels the nerve pathway. Scientists think that each repetition of a signal causes the body to lay down a little more myelin along the axon (or nerve pathway) further insulating it (avoiding energy loss) and making the signal more efficient. In this way the process of laying down more myelin creates a kind of neural superhighway for the behavior signals to travel stronger and faster. Brown et. al. states, "The thickness of the myelin coating correlates with ability, and research strongly suggests that increased practice builds greater myelin along the related pathways, improving the strength and speed of the electrical signals and, as a result, performance." Brown, Roediger, and McDaniel, *Make It Stick*, 1717.

[11]Patricia Cranton, *Understanding and Promoting Transformative Learning: A Guide for Educators of Adults*, 2nd ed. (San Francisco: Jossey-Bass, 2006). Barbara Gross Davis, *Tools for Teaching* (San Francisco: Jossey-Bass, 1993). For helpful tips see chapter eight, "Leading a Discussion," and chapter two, "Sociality," in Joshua R. Eyler, *How Humans Learn: The Science and Stories Behind Effective College Teaching* (Morgantown: West Virginia University Press, 2018).

[12]Hugo Slim and Paul Thompson, *Listening for a Change* (Philadelphia: New Society, 1995), 9.

[13]A worldview can be thought of as both a conscious and subconscious orientation to the world.

[14]"Transformative learning has to do with making meaning out of experiences and questioning assumptions based on prior experience." Cranton, *Understanding and Promoting Transformative Learning*, 8.

[15]"Meaning perspectives are . . . the distinctive ways an individual interprets experience . . . (and) involve criteria for making value judgments and for belief systems." Jack

Mezirow and Associates, *Fostering Critical Reflection in Adults: A Guide to Transformative and Emancipatory Learning* (San Francisco: Jossey-Bass, 1990), 2-3.

[16]Jack Mezirow and Associates, *Learning as Transformation: Critical Perspectives on a Theory in Progress* (San Francisco, Jossey-Bass, 2000), 13-14; Marie-Claire Weinski, Understanding and Promoting Life Change: An Inquiry into the Transformative Learning of Evangelical Theological Students in Germany (Hamburg: Verlag Dr. Kovač, 2006), 38.

[17]Weinski, *Understanding and Promoting Life Change*, 263-64.

[18]Marie-Claire Weinski, "An Inquiry into the Transformative Learning of Evangelical Theological Students in Germany," typed paper (PhD diss. defense summary, Trinity International University, 2006).

[19]Weinski, *Understanding and Promoting Life Change*, 155.

[20]See also Millard Erickson, *Christian Theology*, 2nd ed. (Grand Rapids, MI: Baker, 2007), 1096-97; also Peter C. Craigie, "Priests and Levites," in Walter Elwell, ed., *Baker Encyclopedia of the Bible*, vol. 2 (Grand Rapids, MI: Baker, 1988), 1754-64; also, Skye Jethani, "With God Daily: A Kingdom of Priests," July 26, 2019.

[21]David A. Sousa, *How the Brain Influences Behavior* (New York: Skyhorse Publishing, 2015), 95-97.

[22]Zull, *Brain to Mind*, 288. Italics added.

[23]Zull, *Brain to Mind*, 288.

11. LEARNING TASKS LEADING TO PRACTICE

[1]This example uses a rigged Monopoly game to gather research data. Paul Piff, "Does Money Make You Mean?" filmed October 2013, in San Rafael, CA, TED video, 16:10, www.ted.com/talks/paul_piff_does_money_make_you_mean.

[2]This example gives a way to manipulate a Monopoly game to help learners think about what happens when the rules of engagement are different for different groups. Barb Weidman, "Manipulated Monopoly," Gateway Philadelphia, accessed August 18, 2019, http://sunilsuckoo.github.io/resources/Manipulated%20Monopoly.pdf.

[3]The Ungame now has many subject and age group iterations since it was first created. Today it even has a Christian version with questions about the faith.

[4]The Ted Ward archives offer a helpful guide for debriefing a social system simulation experience to glean helpful insights. Ted Ward, "Debriefing: Converting Experience into Learning," in The Ward Archives, accessed August 17, 2019, www.wardarchives.org /document-archives/simulation-games-and-role-plays/debriefing-converting-experi ences-into-learning/.

[5]J. A. Bowen and C. E. Watson, *Teaching Naked Techniques: A Practical Guide to Designing Better Classes* (San Francisco: Jossey-Bass, 2017), 17.

[6]It was originally published in *A Handbook of Structured Experiences for Human Relations Training*, vol. 1, rev. ed., ed. J. William Pfeiffer and John E. Jones (La Jolla, CA: University Associates, 1974), 25-30. Because it is a simulation that requires complete silence while the simulation is conducted, we have been able to use it in many cultures around the

world, always with the same effective learning results. Online sources for Broken Squares are "Intercultural Activity Toolkit: Broken Squares," NAFSA, February 26, 2009, www .nafsa.org/Professional_Resources/Browse_by_Interest/Internationalizing_Higher _Education/Network_Resources/Teaching,_Learning,_and_Scholarship/Intercultural _Activity_Toolkit__Broken_Squares; "Broken Squares," Building Dynamic Groups Developed by Ohio State University Extension, 2000, www.hunter.cuny.edu/socwork /nrcfcpp/pass/learning-circles/five/Brokensquares.pdf; "Teaching Methods: Broken Squares," Humber, The Center for Teaching and Learning, www.humber.ca/centrefor teachingandlearning/instructional-strategies/teaching-methods/classroom-strategies -designing-instruction/activities-and-games/broken-squares.html.

[7] See www.entrust4.org.

[8] "Facilitator Training," Entrust4, www.entrust4.org/Curriculum/FacilitatorTraining.

[9] Email to authors, December 9, 2018.

[10] See www.entrust4.org.

[11] We recommend Bloom's cognitive taxonomy for more detail in accomplishing this. B. S. Bloom, ed. *Taxonomy of Educational Objectives, Handbook I: The Cognitive Domain.* New York: Longmans, Green, 1956. Another source of revised Bloom is "Revised Bloom's Taxonomy," Iowa State University Center for Excellence in Learning and Teaching, accessed August 18, 2019, www.celt.iastate.edu/teaching/effective-teaching-practices/revised -blooms-taxonomy.

12. Building a Habit

[1] Skye Jethani, "With God Daily: The Danger of a Dis-integrated Life," April 9, 2018.

[2] Vine, W. E. and John R. Kohlenberger II, eds., *The Expanded Vine's Expository Dictionary of New Testament Words.* (Minneapolis, MN: Bethany House Publishers, 1984), 1233-1234.

[3] Greg McKeown, *Essentialism: The Disciplined Pursuit of Less* (New York: Random House, 2014), 209.

[4] Charles Duhigg, *The Power of Habit: Why We Do What We Do in Life and Business* (New York: Random House, 2014), 16-17.

[5] Duhigg, *Power of Habit,* 19.

[6] Duhigg, *Power of Habit,* 51.

[7] Robert M. Sapolsky, *Behave: The Biology of Humans at Our Best and at Our Worst* (New York: Penguin Press, 2017), 70-71.

[8] Duhigg, *Power of Habit,* 25.

[9] James Clear, *Atomic Habits: An Easy and Proven Way to Build Good Habits and Break Bad Ones* (New York: Avery, 2018), 74.

[10] Duhigg, *Power of Habit,* 25.

[11] Roger Steer, *Basic Christian: The Inside Story of John Stott* (Downers Grove, IL: Inter-Varsity Press, 2009), 218.

[12] Discussion with Becky Faber, missionary in Bulgaria.

[13]James E. Zull, *The Art of Changing the Brain: Enriching the Practice of Teaching by Exploring the Biology of Learning* (Sterling, VA: Stylus, 2002), 149.

[14]James E. Zull, *From Brain to Mind: Using Neuroscience to Guide Change in Education* (Sterling, VA: Stylus Publishing, 2011), 173.

[15]Zull, *Brain to Mind*, 174.

[16]Phillippa Lally, et al., "How Habits Are Formed: Modelling Habit Formation in the Real World," *European Journal of Social Psychology* 40, no. 6 (October 2010): 998-1009.

13. Sustaining a Habit

[1]Lauren Villa, "12-Step Drug Addition Recovery Programs," Project Know, accessed August 18, 2019, www.projectknow.com/research/alcoholics-anonymous-12-step/.

[2]Charles Duhigg, *The Power of Habit: Why We Do What We Do in Life and Business* (New York: Random House, 2014), 84.

[3]Duhigg, *Power of Habit*, 84.

[4]Duhigg, *Power of Habit*, 85.

[5]Duhigg, *Power of Habit*, 85.

[6]Duhigg, *Power of Habit*, 100.

[7]Duhigg, *Power of Habit*, 101.

[8]Duhigg, *Power of Habit*, 100.

[9]Duhigg, *Power of Habit*, 109.

[10]David A. Sousa, *How the Brain Learns*, 5th ed. (Thousand Oaks, CA: Corwin, 2017), 98, 137.

[11]Mel Robbins, *The 5 Second Rule: Transform your Life, Work, and Confidence with Everyday Courage* (Brentwood, TN: Savio Republic, 2017), 50.

[12]Lauren Villa, "12-Step Drug Addiction Recovery Programs," *Project Know*, www.projectknow.com/research/alcoholics-anonymous-12-step/.

[13]Duhigg, *Power of Habit*, 85. Italics original.

[14]Sousa, *How the Brain Learns*, 24. See also Timothy Paul Westbrook, "New Reflections on Mirror Neuron Research, the Tower of Babel, and Intercultural Education," *Christian Higher Education* 14:5 (2015): 322-37, https://doi.org/10.1080/15363759.2015.1079749.

[15]Joshua R. Eyler, *How Humans Learn: The Science and Stories Behind Effective College Teaching* (Morgantown: West Virginia University Press, 2018), 69-70.

[16]"Our Church," Saddleback Church, accessed August 19, 2019, https://saddleback.com/visit/about/our-church.

[17]Duhigg, *Power of Habit*, 234.

[18]Charles Duhigg, "How Rick Warren Harnessed the Power of Social Habits," *Christianity Today Online*, August 10, 2012, www.christianitytoday.com/ct/2012/august-web-only/how-rick-warren-harnessed-power-of-social-habits.html. Also quoted in Duhigg, *Power of Habit*, 234.

[19]"Spiritual Maturity," Saddleback Church, https://saddleback.com/learn.

[20]James K. A. Smith, *You Are What You Love: The Spiritual Power of Habit* (Grand Rapids, MI: Brazos Press, 2016), 19. Italics original.

14. FROM HABIT TO CHARACTER

[1]Jan Hábl, quoting Comenius, *Didactica magna*, 70-75, in *Even When No One Is Looking: Fundamental Questions of Ethical Education* (Eugene, OR: Cascade Books, 2018), 102.

[2]Hábl, quoting Comenius, *Pampaedia* II:8, in *Even When No One Is Looking*, 102-3.

[3]Dallas Willard, *The Divine Conspiracy: Rediscovering Our Hidden Life in God* (New York: HarperCollins, 1998), xv.

[4]J. A. Bowen and C. E. Watson, *Teaching Naked Techniques: A Practical Guide to Designing Better Classes* (San Francisco: Jossey-Bass, 2017), 117.

[5]N. T. Wright, *After You Believe: Why Christian Character Matters* (New York: Harper-Collins, 2012), 145.

[6]Note also Col 3:5-10 regarding what we are to "put off."

[7]Wright, *After You Believe*, 151.

[8]Wright, *After You Believe*, 152.

[9]Eric Jensen, *Teaching with the Brain in Mind*, 2nd ed. (Alexandria, VA: Association for Supervision and Curriculum, 2005), 115-18.

Bibliography

Anderson, L. W., and D. R. Krathwohl, eds. *A Taxonomy for Learning, Teaching, and Assessing: A Revision of Bloom's Taxonomy of Educational Objectives.* New York: Longman, 2001.

Andreatta, Britt. *Wired to Grow: Harness the Power of Brain Science to Master Any Skill.* Santa Barbara, CA: Seventh Mind Publishing, 2015.

Ajzen, Icek. "Summary of the TPB [Theory of Planned Behavior] by Ajzen." ValueBased Management.net. Accessed August 20, 2019. www.valuebasedmanagement.net/methods _ajzen_theory_planned_behaviour.html.

Ajzen, Icek, and Dolores Albarracín. "Predicting and Changing Behavior: A Reasoned Action Approach." In *Prediction and Change of Health Behavior: Applying the Reasoned Action Approach,* edited by I. Ajzen, D. Albarracín, and R. Hornik, 3-21. Mahwah, NJ: Lawrence Erlbaum Associates, 2007. www.researchgate.net/publication/261796733_Predicting _and_changing_behavior_A_reasoned_action_approach.

Ajzen, Icek, and Martin Fishbein. "Attitude-Behavior Relations: A Theoretical Analysis and Review of Empirical Research." *Psychological Bulletin* 84 (1977): 888-918.

Backus, William, and Chapian, Marie. *Telling Yourself the Truth: Find Your Way Out of Depression, Anxiety, Fear, Anger, and Other Common Problems by Applying the Principles of Misbelief Therapy.* Bloomington, MN: Bethany House Publishers, 2000.

Bain, Ken. *What the Best College Teachers Do.* Cambridge, MA: Harvard University Press, 2004.

Barclay, William. *Educational Ideals in the Ancient World.* Grand Rapids, MI: Baker, 1959.

Barclay, William. *The Gospel of Luke. The Daily Study Bible.* Edinburgh, UK: The Saint Andrew Press, 1953.

Barclay, William. *The Gospel of Matthew. The Daily Study Bible.* Edinburgh, UK: The Saint Andrew Press, 1957.

Berkhof, Louis. *Systematic Theology,* Part Four, Chapter III, Common Grace, 434-35. Grand Rapids, MI: Eerdmans, 1941.

Berry, Wendell. *Jaber Crow.* Berkeley, CA: Counterpoint, 2001.

Bligh, Donald A. *What's the Use of Lectures?* San Francisco: Jossey-Bass, 2000.

Bloom, B. S., ed. *Taxonomy of Educational Objectives, Handbook I: The Cognitive Domain.* New York: Longmans, Green, 1956.

Bonwell, Charles C., and James A. Eison. *Active Learning: Creating Excitement in the Classroom*. ASHE-ERIC Higher Education Reports, ERIC Clearinghouse on Higher Education. Washington, DC: The George Washington University, School of Education and Human Development, 1991. https://files.eric.ed.gov/fulltext/ED336049.pdf.

Bosler, Annie, and Don Green. "How to Practice Effectively . . . for Just About Anything." TEDEd video. Accessed August 19, 2019. https://ed.ted.com/lessons/how-to-practice -effectively-for-just-about-anything-annie-bosler-and-don-greene.

Bowen, J. A., and C. E. Watson. *Teaching Naked Techniques: A Practical Guide to Designing Better Classes*. San Francisco: Jossey-Bass, 2017.

Brandon, O. R. "Heart." In *Evangelical Dictionary of Theology*, edited by Walter A. Elwell, 499. Grand Rapids, MI: Baker Books, 1984.

Brookfield, S. D. *Becoming a Critically Reflective Teacher*. San Francisco: Jossey-Bass, 1995.

Brown, P. C., H. L. Roediger III, and M. A. McDaniel. *Make It Stick: The Science of Successful Learning*. Cambridge, MA: Belknap Press of Harvard University Press, 2014.

Butler, Katherine J. *Habits of the Heart: 365 Daily Exercises for Living like Jesus*. Carol Stream, IL: Tyndale, 2017.

Calandra, B., A. E. Barron, and I. Thompson-Sellers. "Audio Use in E-learning: What, Why, When, and How?" *International Journal on E-Learning* 7, no. 4 (2008): 589-601.

The Center for Teaching and Learning, Stanford University. "Teaching: How to Create Memorable Lectures." *Speaking of Teaching Newsletter* 14, no. 1 (Winter 2005).

Changing Minds. "Barrier Analysis." ChangingMinds.org. Accessed August 17, 2019. http://changingminds.org/disciplines/change_management/diagnosing_change /barrier_analysis.htm.

Clark, R. C., and R. E. Mayer. *E-learning and the Science of Instruction: Proven Guidelines for Consumers and Designers of Multimedia Learning*. San Francisco: Jossey-Bass, 2003.

Clark, R., F. Nguyen, and J. Sweller. *Efficiency in Learning: Evidence-Based Guidelines to Manage Cognitive Load*. San Francisco: Pfeiffer, 2006.

Clear, James. *Atomic Habits: An Easy and Proven Way to Build Good Habits and Break Bad Ones. Tiny Changes, Remarkable Results*. New York: Avery, 2018.

Craigie, Peter C., "Priests and Levites" in Walter Elwell, ed., *Baker Encyclopedia of the Bible*, vol. 2, 1754-64. Grand Rapids, MI: Baker, 1988.

Cranton, Patricia. *Understanding and Promoting Transformative Learning: A Guide for Educators of Adults*, 2nd ed. San Francisco: Jossey-Bass, 2006.

Dahaene, S. *Reading in the Brain: The Science and Evolution of a Human Invention*. New York: Penguin, 2009.

Daloz, Laurent A. *Effective Teaching and Mentoring: Realizing the Transformational Power of Adult Learning Experiences*. San Francisco: Jossey-Bass, 1986.

Damasio, Antonio. *Descartes' Error*. New York: Harcourt Brace, 1994.

Davis, Barbara Gross. *Tools for Teaching*. San Francisco: Jossey-Bass, 1993.

Davis, Thomas P., Jr. *Barrier Analysis Facilitator's Guide: A Tool for Improving Behavior Change Communication in Child Survival and Community Development Programs*. Washington, DC: Food for the Hungry, 2004.

Dean, Jeremy. *Making Habits, Breaking Habits: Why We Do Things, Why We Don't, and How to Make Any Change Stick.* Philadelphia, PA: Da Capo Press, 2013.

DeLeeuw, K. E., and R. E. Mayer. "A Comparison of Three Measures of Cognitive Load: Evidence for Separable Measures of Intrinsic, Extraneous, and Germane Load." *Journal of Educational Psychology* 100, vol. 1 (2008): 223-34. https://doi.org/10.1037/0022-0663 .100.1.223.

Dennis, Jay. *The Jesus Habits: Exercising the Spiritual Disciplines of Jesus.* Nashville: B&H, 2005.

Deresiewicz, William. *Excellent Sheep: The Miseducation of the American Elite and the Way to a Meaningful Life.* New York: Free Press, 2014.

Dirksen, Julie. *Design for How People Learn,* 2nd ed. San Francisco: New Riders/Peachpit, 2016.

DiSalvo, David. *Brain Changer: How Harnessing Your Brain's Power to Adapt Can Change Your Life.* Dallas: Benbella Books, 2013.

Dolcourt, John. L. "Commitment to Change: A Strategy for Promoting Educational Effectiveness." *Journal of Continuing Education in the Health Profession* 20, vol. 3 (Summer 2000): 156-63.

Doyle, T., and T. Zakrajsek. *The New Science of Learning: How to Learn in Harmony with Your Brain.* Sterling, VA: Stylus, 2013.

Duhigg, Charles. *The Power of Habit: Why We Do What We Do in Life and Business.* New York: Random House, 2014.

Dweck, Carol. *Mindset: The New Psychology of Success.* New York: Ballantine Books, 2017.

Eisner, Elliot W. *The Educational Imagination: On the Design and Evaluation of School Programs,* 2nd ed. New York: Macmillan, 1985.

Elmer, Duane H. "Career Data as Indicators for Curriculum Development in Theological Education." PhD diss., Michigan State University, 1980.

Elmer, Duane H. *Cross-Cultural Servanthood: Serving the World in Christlike Humility.* Downers Grove, IL: InterVarsity Press, 2006.

Entrust. Description of the module *Facilitating Relational Learning (FRL).* www.entrust4 .org/facilitator-training.

Erickson, Millard. "The Government of the Church." in *Christian Theology,* 2nd ed., 1096-97. Grand Rapids, MI: Baker, 2007.

Eyler, Joshua R. *How Humans Learn: The Science and Stories Behind Effective College Teaching.* Morgantown: West Virginia University Press, 2018.

Ezigbo, Victor I. "Rethinking the Sources of African Contextual Christology." *Journal of Theology for Southern Africa* 32 (2008): 53-70.

Fink, L. D. *Creating Significant Learning Experiences: An Integrated Approach to Designing College Courses,* 2nd ed. San Francisco, CA: Jossey-Bass, 2013.

Fishbein, M., and I. Ajzen. *Belief, Attitude, Intention, and Behavior: An Introduction to Theory and Research.* Reading, MA: Addison-Wesley, 1975.

Fishbein, M., H. C. Triandis, F. H. Kanfer, M. Becker, S. E. Middlestadt, and A. Eichler. "Factors Influencing Behavior and Behavior Change." In *Handbook of Health Psychology,* edited by A. Baum, T. A. Revenson, and J. E. Singer, 3-17. Mahwah, NJ: Erlbaum, 2001.

Fowler, James W. *Faith Development and Pastoral Care.* Philadelphia, PA: Fortress Press, 1986.

Frederick, Peter J. "Engaging Students Actively in Large Lecture Settings." In Christine A. Stanley and M. Erin Porter. *Engaging Large Lecture Classes: Strategies and Techniques for College Faculty*, 58-66. Bolton, MA: Anker Publishing, 2002.

Gallup. "2015 Gallup Student Poll Results." Accessed August 17, 2019. https://news.gallup .com/reports/189926/student-poll-2015-results.aspx.

Gardner, Howard. Foreword to *Emotions, Learning and the Brain: Embodied Brains, Social Minds, and the Art of Learning* by Mary Helen Immordino-Yang, 7-10. New York: Norton, 2015.

Global Learning Partners, Inc. Accessed August 20, 2019. www.globallearningpartners.com.

Hábl, Jan. *Even When No One Is Looking: Fundamental Questions of Ethical Education.* Eugene, OR: Cascade Books, 2018.

Hart, Carl L. *High Price: A Neuroscientist's Journey to Self-Discovery that Challenges Everything You Know about Drugs and Society.* New York: Harper, 2013.

Hodge, David. "Piaget's Equilibration, One Side of the Coin?" *Christian Education Journal* XV, no. 2 (Winter 1995): 40-44.

Hoffeld, David. "Want to Know What Your Brain Does When It Hears a Question?" February 21, 2017. Fast Company. www.fastcompany.com/3068341/want-to-know-what -your-brain-does-when-it-hears-a-question.

Holtrop, Philip. "A Strange Language Toward a Biblical Conception of Truths and a New Mood for Doing Reformed Theology." *Reformed Journal* 27, no. 2 (February 1977): 9-13.

Howe, Reuel. *The Miracle of Dialogue.* Minneapolis, MN: Seabury Press, 1963.

Hunter, James Davison. *The Death of Character: Moral Education in an Age Without Good or Evil.* New York: Basic Books, 2000.

Immordino-Yang, Mary Helen. *Emotions, Learning, and the Brain: Embodied Brains, Social Minds, and the Art of Learning.* New York: Norton, 2015.

Immordino-Yang, Mary Helen, and Creativity Institute and Rossier School of Education. "Implications of Affective and Social Neuroscience for Educational Theory." *Educational Philosophy and Theory* 43, no. 1 (2011): 98-103.

Immordino-Yang, Mary Helen, and Matthias Faeth. "The Role of Emotion and Skilled Intuition in Learning." In *Mind, Brain, and Education: Neuroscience Implications for the Classroom*, edited by David A. Sousa, 69-84. Bloomington, IN: Solution Tree Press, 2010.

Iowa State University. "Revised Bloom's Taxonomy." Iowa State University Center for Excellence in Learning and Teaching. Accessed 18 August 2019, www.celt.iastate.edu /teaching/effective-teaching-practices/revised-blooms-taxonomy.

Jarrett, Christian. "What Are We Like? 10 Psychology Findings That Reveal the Worst of Human Nature." The British Psychological Society, *Research Digest* (blog). October 12, 2018. https://digest.bps.org.uk/2018/10/12/what-are-we-like-10-psychology-findings-that -reveal-the-worst-of-human-nature/.

Jensen, Eric. *Brain-Based Learning: A New Paradigm of Teaching*, 2nd ed. Thousand Oaks, CA: Corwin, 2008.

Jensen, Eric. "Seven Ways to Thrive During Overload." Jensen Learning blog. Accessed August 20, 2019. www.jensenlearning.com/7-ways-to-thrive-during-overload/.

Jensen, Eric. *Teaching with the Brain in Mind,* 2nd ed. Alexandria, VA: Association for Supervision and Curriculum, 2005.

Jethani, Skye. "With God Daily: The Danger of a Dis-integrated Life." April 9, 2018. dailydevotional@skyejethani.com.

Jethani, Skye. "With God Daily: How to Not Fear Cognitive Dissonance." November 20, 2017. dailydevotional@skyejethani.com.

Jethani, Skye. "With God Daily: A Kingdom of Priests." July 26, 2019. dailydevotional@skyejethani.com.

Johnson, George. *In the Palaces of Memory: How We Build the World Inside Our Heads.* New York: Penguin Random House, 1992.

Kagan, Jerome M. *Galen's Prophecy.* New York: Basic Books, 1994.

Kegan, R., and L. L. Lahey. *Immunity to Change: How to Overcome It and Unlock the Potential in Yourself and Your Organization.* Boston: Harvard Business Review Press, 2009.

Kittle, Bonnie. *A Practical Guide to Conducting a Barrier Analysis*, 2nd ed. New York: Helen Keller International, 2017.

Knoblauch, Neil. "On Becoming: Between Statues and Clay." *Spore, tussen klippe en wolke* (blog). November 8, 2018. https://nielknoblauch.wordpress.com/2018/11/08/on-becoming -between-statues-clay/#more-628.

Kolb, David. *Experiential Learning: Experience as the Source of Learning and Development.* Englewood Cliffs, NJ: Prentice Hall, 1984.

Krathwohl, D. R., B. S. Bloom, and B. B. Masia. *Taxonomy of Educational Objectives, Handbook II: Affective Domain.* New York: David McKay, 1964.

Kuh, G. D., J. Kinzie, J. H. Schuh, and J. H. Whitt. *Assessing Conditions to Enhance Educational Effectiveness: The Inventory for Student Engagement and Success.* San Francisco, CA: Jossey-Bass, 2005.

Lally, Phillippa, Cornelia H. M. van Jaarsveld, Henry W. W. Potts, and Jane Wardle. "How Habits Are Formed: Modelling Habit Formation in the Real World." *European Journal of Social Psychology* 40, no. 6 (October 2010): 998-1009.

Lewis, C. S. "The Weight of Glory." In *The Essential C. S. Lewis,* ed. Lyle W. Dorsett, 366-70. New York: Collier, 1988.

Luciani, Joseph. "Why 80 Percent of New Year's Resolutions Fail." *U.S. News & World Report,* December 29, 2015. https://health.usnews.com/health-news/blogs/eat-run/articles /2015-12-29/why-80-percent-of-new-years-resolutions-fail.

Maddix, Mark A and Blevins, Dean Gray. *Neuroscience and Christian Formation.* Charlotte, NC: Information Age, 2017.

Major, Claire Howell, Michael S. Harris, and Todd Zakrajsek. *Teaching for Learning: 101 Intentionally Designed Educational Activities to Put Students on the Path to Success.* New York: Routledge, 2016.

Maltz, Maxwell. *Psycho-Cybernetics,* 1st ed. New York: Simon & Schuster, 1960.

McEachan, R., N. Taylor, R. Harrison, R. Lawton, P. Gardner, and M. Conner. "Meta-Analysis of the Reasoned Action Approach (RAA) to Understanding Health Behaviors." *Annals of Behavioral Medicine* 50, no. 4 (May 2016). https://doi.org/10.1007/s12160-016-9798-4.

McGonigal, J. "Gaming Can Make a Better World." Filmed February 2010 in Long Beach, CA. TED talk. 19:36. www.ted.com/talks/jane_mcgonigal_gaming_can_make_a_better _world.html.

McGuire, S. *Teach Students How to Learn: Strategies You Can Incorporate into Any Course to Improve Student Metacognition, Study Skills, and Motivation.* Sterling, VA: Stylus, 2015.

McKeachie, Wilbert J., Nancy Chism, Robert Menges, Marilla Svinicki, and Claire Ellen Weinstein. *Teaching Tips: Strategies, Research, and Theory for College and University Teachers*, 9th ed. Lexington, MA: D. C. Heath, 1994.

McKeown, Greg. *Essentialism: The Disciplined Pursuit of Less.* New York: Random House, 2014.

McLeod, Saul. "Cognitive Dissonance," *Simply Psychology* (blog). February 5, 2018. www .simplypsychology.org/cognitive-dissonance.html.

Medina, John. *Brain Rules for Aging Well: 10 Principles for Staying Vital, Happy and Sharp.* Seattle: Pear Press, 2017.

Medina, John. *Brain Rules: Twelve Principles for Surviving and Thriving at Work, Home and School*, 2nd ed. Seattle: Pear Press, 2014.

Mednick, S. C., K. Nakayama, J. L. Cantero, M. Atienza, A. A. Levin, N. Pathak, and R. Stickgold. "The Restorative Effect of Naps on Perceptual Deterioration." *Nature Neuroscience* 5, no. 7 (July 2002): 677-81.

Mezirow, Jack, and Associates. *Fostering Critical Reflection in Adults: A Guide to Transformative and Emancipatory Learning.* San Francisco: Jossey-Bass, 1990.

Mezirow, Jack, and Associates. *Learning as Transformation: Critical Perspectives on a Theory in Progress.* San Francisco: Jossey-Bass, 2000.

Mezirow, Jack. *Transformative Dimensions of Adult Learning.* San Francisco: Jossey-Bass, 1991.

Mezirow, Jack. "Transformative Learning: Theory to Practice." *New Directions in Adult and Continuing Education. Insights from Practice* 74 (Summer 1997): 5-12.

Miller, G. A. "The Magical Number Seven, Plus or Minus Two: Some Limits on Our Capacity to Process Information." *Psychological Review* 63, no. 2 (1956): 81-97. https://doi.org /10.1037/h0043158.

Moreno, R., and R. Mayer. "Interactive Multimodal Learning Environments." *Educational Psychology Review* 19 (2007): 309-26.

Mousavi, S., R. Low, and J. Sweller. "Reducing Cognitive Load by Mixing Auditory and Visual Presentation Modes." *Journal of Educational* Psychology 87, no. 2 (1995): 319-34. doi:10.1037/0022-0663.87.2.319.

Neal, David T., Wendy Wood, and Jeffrey M. Quinn. "Habit: A Repeat Performance." *Current Directions in Psychological Science* 15, no. 4 (2006): 198-202.

Newberg, Andrew, and Mark Robert Waldman. *How God Changes Your Brain: Breakthrough Findings from a Leading Neuroscientist.* New York: Ballantine Books, 2009.

Nilson, Linda B. *Teaching at Its Best: A Research-Based Resource for College Instructors*. San Francisco: Jossey-Bass, 2006.

Novak, J. D., and A. J. Cañas. *The Theory Underlying Concept Maps and How to Construct Them*. Pensacola: Florida Institute for Human and Machine Cognition, 2008. http://cmap.ihmc.us/Publications/ResearchPapers/TheoryUnderlyingConceptMaps.pdf.

Paas, Fred, Heerlen Alexander Renkl, and John Sweller. "Cognitive Load Theory and Instructional Design: Recent Developments." *Educational Psychologist* 38, no. 1 (2003): 1-4. https://doi.org/10.1207/S15326985EP3801_1.

Palmer, Parker. *The Courage to Teach: Exploring the Inner Landscape of a Teacher's Life*. San Francisco: Jossey-Bass, 2017.

Palmer, Parker. *A Hidden Wholeness: The Journey Toward an Undivided Life*. San Francisco: Jossey-Bass, 2009.

Palmer, Parker. *To Know as We Are Known: Education as a Spiritual Journey*. San Francisco: HarperCollins, 1993.

Pajares, F. "William James: Our Father Who Begat Us." In *Educational Psychology: A Century of Contributions*, edited by B. J. Zimmerman and D. H. Schunk, 41-64. Mahwah, NJ: Erlbaum, 2003.

Pashler, H., M. McDaniel, D. Rohrer, and R. Bjork. "Learning Styles: Concepts and Evidence." *Psychological Science in the Public Interest* 9, no. 3 (2008): 105-109.

Pavio, A. "Dual Coding Theory: Retrospect and Current Status." *Canadian Journal of Psychology* 45 (1991): 255-87.

Pawlak, R., A. M. Magarinos, J. Melchor, B. McEwen, and S. Strickland. "Tissue Plasminogen Activator in the Amygdala Is Critical for Stress-Induced Anxiety-Like Behavior." *Nature Neuroscience* 6 (January 2003): 168-74.

Pearcey, Nancy. *Finding Truth: 5 Principles for Unmasking Atheism, Secularism and Other God Substitutes*. Colorado Springs, CO: David C. Cook, 2015.

Penner, Peter F., ed. *Theological Education as Mission*. Schwarzenfeld, Germany: Neufeld Verlag, 2005.

Pfeiffer, J. William, and John E. Jones, eds. *A Handbook of Structured Experiences for Human Relations Training, vol. 1*, rev. ed. La Jolla, CA: University Associates, 1974. 25-30.

Ping, Raedy, and Susan Goldin-Meadow. "Gesturing Saves Cognitive Resources When Talking About Nonpresent Objects." *Cognitive Science* 34, no.4 (2010): 602-19. https://doi.org/10.1111/j.1551-6709.2010.01102.

Plass, Jan L., Slava Kalyuga, and Detlev Leutner. "Individual Differences and Cognitive Load Theory." In *Cognitive Load Theory*, edited by Jan Plass, Roxana Moreno, and Roland Brunken, 65-90. Cambridge: Cambridge University Press, 2010.

Plato. *The Republic*. Translated by B. Jowett. Thousand Oaks, CA: BN Publishing, 2009.

Prochaska, James O., Carlos C. DiClemente, and John C. Norcross. "In Search of How People Change: Applications to Addictive Behavior." *American Psychologist* 47, no. 9 (September 1992): 1102-14. https://doi.org/10.3109/10884609309149692.

Prochaska, James O., J. C. Prochaska, and John C. Norcross. "Stages of Change." *Psychotherapy* 38, no. 4 (Winter 2001): 443-48.

Prochaska, James O., et al. "Stages of Change and Provisional Balance for 12 Problem Behaviors." *Health Psychology* 13, no.1 (1994): 39-46.

Richards, Lawrence O. *A Theology of Christian Education*, 71. Grand Rapids, MI: Zondervan, 1975.

Richards, J. P., and C. B. McCormick. "Effective Interspersed Conceptual Pre-questions on Note-taking in Listening Comprehension." *Journal of Educational Psychology* 80 (1988): 592-94.

Rigsby, Rick. *Lessons from a Third Grade Dropout: How the Timeless Wisdom of One Man Can Impact an Entire Generation*. Nashville, TN: Thomas Nelson, 2006.

Rigsby, Rick. "The Wisdom of a Third Grade Dropout Will Change Your Life." Speech on video, 10:21. www.youtube.com/watch?v=Bg_Q7KYWG1g.

Robbins, Mel. *The 5 Second Rule: Transform Your Life, Work, and Confidence with Everyday Courage*. Brentwood, TN: Savio Republic, 2017.

Robinson, Ken. *The Element: How Finding Your Passion Changes Everything*. New York: Penguin Books, 2009.

Robinson, M. D., E. R. Watkins, and E. Harmon-Jones, eds. *Handbook of Cognition and Emotion*. New York: Guilford Press, 2013.

Saddleback Church. https://saddleback.com/.

Sana, F., T. Weston, and N. J. Cepeda. "Laptop Multitasking Hinders Classroom Learning for Both Users and Nearby Peers." *Computers and Education* 62 (2013): 24-31. https://doi.org/10.1016/j.compedu.2012.10.003.

Sanes, J., and J. Lichtman. "Induction, Assembly, Maturation, and Maintenance of a Post-synaptic Apparatus." *Nature Reviews Neuroscience* 2, no.11 (November 2001): 791-805.

Sapolsky, Robert M. *Behave: The Biology of Humans at Our Best and at Our Worst*. New York: Penguin, 2017.

Schenck, Jeb, and Jessie Cruickshank. "Evolving Kolb: Experiential Education in the Age of Neuroscience." *Journal of Experiential Education* 38, no.1 (2015): 73-95.

Schön, D. A. *The Reflective Practitioner: How Professionals Think in Action*. New York: Basic Books, 1984.

Schroth, M. L. "The Effects of Delay of Feedback on a Delayed Concept Formation Transfer Task." *Contemporary Educational Psychology* 17 (1992): 78-82.

Seamands, David A. *Healing for Damaged Emotions*. Colorado Springs, CO: David C. Cook, 2015.

Shams, L., and A. R. Seitz. "Benefits of Multisensory Learning." *Trends in Cognitive Sciences* 12, no. 11 (2008): 411-17.

Smilkstein, Rita. *We're Born to Learn: Using the Brain's Natural Learning Process to Create Today's Curriculum*, 2nd ed. Thousand Oaks, CA: Corwin, 2011.

Smith, James K.A. *You Are What You Love: The Spiritual Power of Habit*. Grand Rapids, MI: Brazos Press, 2016.

Slavin, Robert E. "Student Characteristics, Practice and Achievement in Physical Education." *Journal of Educational Research* 21, no. 2 (1994): 54-61.

Slim, Hugo, and Paul Thompson. *Listening for a Change.* Philadelphia: New Society, 1995.

Sousa, David A. *How the Brain Influences Behavior: Strategies for Managing K-12 Classrooms.* New York: Skyhorse Publishing, 2015. First published 2009 by Corwin (Thousand Oaks, CA).

Sousa, David A. *How the Brain Learns,* 5th ed. Thousand Oaks, CA: Corwin, 2017.

Sousa, David A., ed. *Mind, Brain, and Education: Neuroscience Implications for the Classroom.* Bloomington, IN: Solution Tree Press, 2010.

Steer, Roger. *Basic Christian: The Inside Story of John Stott.* Downers Grove, IL: InterVarsity Press, 2010.

Strobel, Kyle. *Metamorpha: Jesus as a Way of Life.* Grand Rapids, MI: Baker, 2007.

Stuart, J. "Medical Student Concentration During Lectures." *Lancet* 312, no. 8088 (September 1978): 514-16.

Sylwester, Robert. "Unconscious Emotions." *Educational Leadership* 58, no. 3 (November 2000): 20-24.

Tolstoy, Leo. *Path of Life.* Translated by Maureen Cote, 214. New York: Nova Science, 2002.

Vanhoozer, Kevin J. "'One Rule to Rule Them All?' Theological Method in an Era of World Christianity." In *Globalizing Theology: Belief and Practice in an Era of World Christianity,* edited by Craig Ott and Harold Netland, 85-126. Grand Rapids, MI: Baker Academic, 2006.

Vella, Jane. *Learning to Listen, Learning to Teach.* San Francisco: Jossey-Bass, 2002.

Vella, Jane. *Taking Learning to Task.* San Francisco: Jossey-Bass, 2000.

Vella, Jane. *Training Through Dialogue.* San Francisco: Jossey-Bass, 1995.

Villa, Lauren. "12-Step Drug Addiction Recovery Programs." Project Know. www.projectknow.com/research/alcoholics-anonymous-12-step/.

Vine, W. E. *The Expanded Vine's Expository Dictionary of New Testament Words.* Edited by John R. Kohlenberger III. Minneapolis, MN: Bethany House Publishers, 1984.

Ward, Ted. *The Ward Archives.* "A Role Play: A Community Learning Activity." Accessed August 20, 2019. www.wardarchives.org/document-archives/simulation-games-and-role-plays/role-play-community-learning-activity/.

Warren, Rick. *The Purpose Driven Life: What on Earth Am I Here For?* Grand Rapids, MI: Zondervan, 2002.

Weimer, Maryellen. *Learner-Centered Teaching.* San Francisco: Jossey-Bass, 2002.

Weinski, Marie-Claire. "An Inquiry into the Transformative Learning of Evangelical Theological Students in Germany." PhD diss., Trinity International University, 2006, www.researchgate.net/publication/34179721_An_inquiry_into_the_transformative_learning_of_evangelical_theological_students_in_Germany.

Weinski, Marie-Claire. *Understanding and Promoting Life Change: An Inquiry into the Transformative Learning of Evangelical Theological Students in Germany.* Hamburg: Verlag Dr. Kovač, 2006.

Willard, Dallas. *The Divine Conspiracy: Rediscovering Our Hidden Life in God.* New York: HarperCollins, 1998.

Willis, Judy. "The Current Impact of Neuroscience on Teaching and Learning." In *Mind, Brain, and Education: Neuroscience Implications for the Classroom*, edited by David A. Sousa, 45-68. Bloomington, IN: Solution Tree Press, 2010.

Willhelm, I., S. Diekelmann, I. Molzow, A. Ayoub, M. Mölle, and J. Born. "Sleep Selectively Enhances Memory Expected to Be of Future Relevance." *Journal of Neuroscience* 31 (2011): 1563-69. https://doi.org/10.1523/JNEUROSCI.3575-10.2011.

Winkelms, M. A. "Transparency in Teaching: Faculty Share Data and Improve Students' Learning." *Liberal Education* 99, no. 2 (Spring 2013). www.aacu.org/publications-research /periodicals/transparency-teaching-faculty-share-data-and-improve-students.

Wiske, Martha Stone, ed. *Teaching for Understanding: Linking Research with Practice*. San Francisco: Jossey-Bass, 1998.

Wiske, Martha Stone. "What Is Teaching for Understanding?" In *Teaching for Understanding: Linking Research with Practice*, edited by Martha Stone Wiske, 72. San Francisco: Jossey-Bass, 2000.

Wright, N. T. *After You Believe: Why Christian Character Matters*. New York: Harper-Collins, 2012.

Zull, J. E. *The Art of Changing the Brain: Enriching the Practice of Teaching by Exploring the Biology of Learning*. Sterling, VA: Stylus, 2002.

Zull, J. E. *From Brain to Mind: Using Neuroscience to Guide Change in Education*. Sterling, VA: Stylus, 2011.

Author and Subject Index

Scripture Index

Also by Duane Elmer

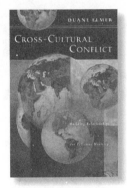 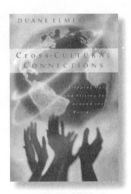 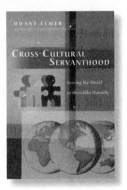

Cross-Cultural Conflict
978-0-8308-1657-6

Cross-Cultural Connections
978-0-8308-2309-3

Cross-Cultural Servanthood
978-0-8308-3378-8

Finding the Textbook You Need

The IVP Academic Textbook Selector
is an online tool for instantly finding the IVP books
suitable for over 250 courses across 24 disciplines.

ivpacademic.com